D1132730

SURVIVING IN THE HOUR OF DARKNESS

Surviving in the Hour of Darkness

THE HEALTH AND WELLNESS OF WOMEN OF COLOUR AND INDIGENOUS WOMEN

Edited by G. Sophie Harding

UNIVERSITY OF
CALGARY
PRESS

JUN 0 3 2005

DOUGLAS COLLEGE LIBRARY

© 2005 by G. Sophie Harding

Published by the
University of Calgary Press
2500 University Drive NW
Calgary, Alberta, Canada T2N 1N4
www.uofcpress.com

No part of this publication may be
reproduced, stored in a retrieval
system or transmitted, in any form
or by any means, without the prior
written consent of the publisher or a
licence from The Canadian Copyright
Licensing Agency (Access Copyright).
For an Access Copyright licence, visit
www.accesscopyright.ca or call toll
free to 1-800-893-5777.

We acknowledge the financial
support of the Government of Canada,
through the Book Publishing Industry
Development Program (BPIDP),
and the Alberta Foundation for the
Arts for our publishing activities. We
acknowledge the support of the Canada
Council for the Arts for our publishing
program.

COMMITTED TO THE DEVELOPMENT OF CULTURE AND THE ARTS

Canada Council   Conseil des Arts
for the Arts   du Canada

LIBRARY AND ARCHIVES CANADA
CATALOGUING IN PUBLICATION

Surviving in the hour of darkness : the
health and wellness of women
of colour and indigenous women /
edited by G. Sophie Harding.

Includes bibliographical references and
index.
ISBN 1-55238-101-3

1. Minority women—Medical care—
Canada.   2. Indian women—Medical
care—Canada.   3. Minority women
—Health and hygiene—Canada.
4. Indian women—Health and
hygiene—Canada.   I. Harding, G.
Sophie, 1970–

RA564.86.S87 2005   362.1'089'0097
C2004-907365-6

Cover design, Mieka West.
Internal design & typesetting,
zijn digital

This book is printed on acid-free paper.

Printed and bound in Canada by
Houghton Boston.

for my mother

Thank you for the years of
wholesome soups, well-packed lunches,
home-cooked meals and worrying about my wellness.
You are the woman I aspire to be.

Contents

Acknowledgments

This book was not an easy journey. Thanks to everyone who made it possible. My love and blessings to the following: To organizations such as Women's Health in Women's Hands that went the extra mile in the production of this book, a very special thanks to Notisha Massaquoi and Linda Cornwell for their tremendous faith and support. To all the people who submitted their work, thank you for your stories and dedication to wellness. To all the people who supported this book by getting the word out there, every raindrop contributes to filling the ocean. Thanks to the University of Calgary Press for recognizing the importance of publishing this anthology. I give my thanks and eternal gratitude to my family and friends for their continuous support and encouragement throughout the years. To my mother, who is also my best friend – if I took two lifetimes to say thank you for everything it still wouldn't be enough. To my husband, just in case I forget to tell you – you are the dream I never dreamt, the wish I never made, the song I never wrote, the unexpected pot of gold at the end of the rainbow. Thanks for some of the best times of my life. I thank God, who holds the key to my wellness and health. To all women who fight illness everyday, keep on keeping on, the struggle continues.

– Sophie

Photo/Art Gallery Acknowledgments

The photos and artwork in this anthology serve as a medium to express diverse thoughts, ideas, and sounds. A very special thanks to the following people for lending their artistic talents to this book:

TROY HUNTER, thank you for sharing your Aunt Patsy's story; through your lens we come to know her. (Pages 184, 193)

SORAYA PEERBAYE, I really enjoy your pictures – you truly capture the spirit of the Women's Health in Women's Hands Rooftop Gardeners. (Pages 274, 275, 276)

ROXANE TRACEY, you are a very talented woman and your work inspires those who come in contact with it. Thank you for sharing your poetic artwork. (*Her Spirit* – page 1, *One* – page 32, *Her Many Faces* – Page 123, *US* – page 301)

www.poeticartgallery.com

Foreword

Sometime during the 1980s, Women of Colour around the world decided that we were sick and tired of being sick and tired. Women started telling stories filled with pain, laughter, insight and new information. As we talked with each other, we came to understand the interlocking effects of race, sex, and class on our health. It is no accident that women of color have the worst health statistics. We have come to understand that racism in the health care system not only unjustly affects the delivery of care, but racism also has a negative impact on our personal health. Many of us had feelings of isolation and alienation that kept us from talking to each other and recognizing our inner truths about our lives.

The telling of our life stories is one of the most powerful mediums that we can use for self-analysis. As we start to share openly in the presence of others, we are able to distinguish our actions from those of an oppressive society. When we hear each other's stories, we are able to draw from our sisters' personal experiences, make comparisons to our own life and develop a way to address our problems more effectively. Recognizing our truths represents the first step toward personal liberation.

Surviving in the Hour of Darkness is a journey into health and healing, as women tell us in detail how racism penetrates the health care system and compromises our health and well-being. This book provides an opportunity to closely examine health issues within a cultural context. A lack of access to adequate health care is a theme that runs through the stories of most Women of Colour. Our inability to achieve ongoing preventative services means that our poor health status today spells doom for many generations to come.

Health and wellness is reflective of the interlocking factors of physical, emotional and spiritual well-being. The sharing that women offer in *Surviving in the Hour of Darkness* reflects the strength and resiliency of women's power to obtain and maintain optimal health, in spite of barriers that oppress and marginalize us.

These women are no longer in the dark. Their stories light the way for themselves and for us to fight harder for the most fundamental of all human rights – a sensitive health care delivery system. Our struggle unites us!

A luta continua,
Byllye Y. Avery

Preface: On Our Way to Recovery

I write this book not as a destination but as the beginning of a long and essential journey. The health and wellness of Women of Colour and Indigenous Women encompasses the social, economic, cultural, ideological, and political arenas of a given society. While this anthology focuses mainly on Canada, some papers come from other countries. This book offers an insight and serves as the beginning of a discussion that will hopefully encourage health care officials, women, educators, policy makers, academics and all those wanting to understand the many factors that impact health and wellness. This endeavour is hard to accomplish; first, because we all speak different languages, and second, because we have different perceptions of what wellness is. In putting together a book of this nature, how we define ourselves as women comes into question. I use the expression Women of Colour and Indigenous Women to represent some of the marginalized and the disenfranchised in our society. "Women of Colour and Indigenous Women" covers many people. Unfortunately, we cannot touch on all illnesses, issues, solutions, and problems that our vast communities face on a daily basis. Through the voices of many women this anthology enables us to bring to the forefront some of the issues affecting Women of Colour and Indigenous Women; perhaps then we can begin to build health care systems, attitudes, and policies that encircle and embody some of the health concerns of these women.

For years, Women of Colour and Indigenous Women have been saying to the liberal White Western feminist movement that we do not all fall under one umbrella called "WOMAN," with the same concerns, ideas, and ways of defining ourselves. These are the same arguments that come to the foreground when looking at health research and its impact on Women of Colour and Indigenous Women, as outlined in the report "What Women Prescribe: Report and Recommendations": "The lack of research data for Aboriginal women, women with disabilities, women of colour, older women, and lesbians, on a whole range of health issues is striking. Just as traditional research has been dominated by white men, feminist research has been dominated by middle-class, non-disabled women."[1] In looking at Indigenous and Women of Colour communities there is little or no information available which examines and identifies their specific concerns and issues with regard to health and wellness. For example, in Vancouver, British Columbia, the little research that has been done illustrates that Aboriginal women face many systemic barriers that keep them from accessing crucial health care resources that are essential in maintaining good health, such as mammograms and pap smears. These systemic barriers include having to deal with a health care system that does not have a good grasp or understanding of their cultural beliefs, practices, and values. Unfortunately, these findings have not made an impact on policy making with respect to Aboriginal women and health.[2]

In order for society to understand the health concerns that the diverse communities of Indigenous Women and Women of Colour face, it is imperative to examine areas such as history (this includes migration and immigration), socio-economic factors, cultural diversity, gender, race, and class. We have to analyze how and what these factors contribute to women achieving a good state of health and wellness. Only then can society start to combat illness and promote health and wellness. We cannot begin to change our heath care system unless we discuss, deconstruct, and re-examine the aforementioned factors that exist on the outskirts of our health care system, factors that shape and inform women's lives and women's very existences.[3]

Women of Colour and Indigenous Women face inaccessibility and lack of availability in the health care system. Lack of funding for these communities of women results in misinformation and miscommunication and can sometimes result in health care delivery being gender-biased and racist. Deficient funding can impede access to some basic services; for example, in Nova Scotia lack of funding has been a contributing factor to many Black communities having little access to transportation. This has been a disincentive for people wanting to get to health care centres and acquire the information and treatment that they need. Regrettably, because of this, many Black people die or remain sick with illness and diseases that could have been treated and/or prevented.[4] Communication and understanding is essential between health care workers and the women that they are treating. For example, many new immigrants face language barriers and culture shock – a bombardment with different social customs and feelings of isolation that comes with resettling in a different country. These factors can absolutely impact health and wellness for these women and should be addressed in consultations.[5]

This anthology illustrates, through the voices of many women, that health care workers cannot begin to solve the problems associated with achieving wellness for Women of Colour and Indigenous Women without an extensive dialogue with the women they are treating. There needs to be an understanding of who we are and where we're coming from. As a society we must identify and recognize the barriers, in order to break them down and make progress in health care. There are several recommendations that would aid in the development of policies and procedures in health care practices for Women of Colour and Indigenous Women: any holistic definition of health and wellness should include the influence of cultural background, socio-economic conditions, gender, class, psychological issues, and history; research involving Indigenous Women and Women of Colour communities should take into consideration the impact of relocation and immigration on health and wellness; and finally, a spirit of collectivity and a dialogue with members in various communities is essential as it aids in the understanding of cultural beliefs and values.[6]

Endnotes

1 *What Women Prescribe.* Report and recommendations from the national symposium, "Women in Partnership: Working towards Inclusive, Gender-Sensitive Health Policies," Canadian Advisory Council on the Status of Women, May 1995.

2 *Marginalized Voices from the Downtown Eastside: Aboriginal Women Speak about Their Health Experiences* (National Network on Environments and Women's Health, March 1, 2001), 1.

3 Joan Gilmour and Dianne Martin, *Women's Poverty, Women's Health: The Role of Access to Justice*, September 2001.

4 *Racism as a Determinant of Women's Health: A Workshop by Susan Edmonds*, presented in two locations on September 17, 2001 (York University & Women's Health in Women's Hands), 5.

5 *Promoting the Health and Well Being of South Asian Women: A Health Promotion Project* (South Asian Community and Region of Peel Health Department, Winter 1999) 6.

6 Ibid., 31.

Introduction

My aim in this book is to advance the understanding of factors that contribute to the health and wellness of Women of Colour and Indigenous Women. This anthology is a resource that can be used in a wide variety of venues, including schools and health care settings. The principles upon which I built this anthology are well summarized as follows: (1) As a society we need to realize that there are many different ways to know and understand what is wellness and what it means to be healthy; (2) Cultural background, class, religious belief systems, and economic conditions impact and inform the way people communicate and convey who they are and what they need; (3) It is essential to listen to and understand women's personal stories and testimonies told in their own voices; (4) We must as a society deconstruct the barriers that pose threats to the physical, emotional, and spiritual health and well being of women; (5) Indigenous and Women of Colour community members should be active participants in health research and policy making.[1]

This book is divided into two sections: (1) *Perspectives on Health in the Diaspora: Understanding the Challenges*, and (2) *Her-story: Living with Illness*. The first section addresses some of the systemic barriers within society that hamper the health and wellness of Women of Colour and Indigenous Women. In the second section, women, through poetry, prose, and essays find different ways to express thoughts and struggles with their illnesses. This section looks at how women are surviving with sickness. When you live on the margins of society, you do what you can to make the margins work for you. Strategies for coping with illness differ from woman to woman and from community to community. The conception of health and wellness and what it means to be healthy also differs from woman to woman and from community to community. For example, many people within the health care industry tend to define health in terms of body weight, body size, family history or in terms of being disease-free or not having a specific identifiable illness. A British survey indicates that many people associate having good health with being emotionally firm, having a high energy level, and the ability to complete a multiplicity of activities.[2]

I take my hat off to all women who are living with and fighting to overcome various kinds of illness. Traditionally, Women of Colour and Indigenous Women find their own ways to exist outside the health care system. Some of us find comfort in our families, friends, in God, and in holistic forms of health practices that help us to overcome whatever illness we are facing. Many women define being "healthy" as encompassing all aspects of the spirit, mind, body, and heart. To be truly well, one must achieve oneness and balance, uniting all aspects of the self. The road to wellness is not easy. Many women fail and many of us succeed. I think the key is to establish foundations that enable us to talk about our experiences in an open and honest way.

During the course of a day, we hear stories about women who are sick or have died; they remain nameless and faceless. Too many women face their illnesses alone and die without their stories being told. Many women feel that no one understands or cares. Loneliness, depression, and fear plague the lives of too many women. It is time to speak and listen, to hear and be heard. Perhaps in sharing our experiences and walking in each other's shoes we can gain wisdom, compassion, and understanding. Women of Colour and Indigenous women have learned that we must challenge the status quo. Women are breaking down the barriers and attempting to find solutions to their health issues. It is necessary to focus on the future, to make room where there is none. Advocacy and resistance have become a necessary part of our existence. It is imperative that we let our voices be heard. It is a question of silence equalling death or resistance equalling life. Our health care workers, those who give us medications, diagnoses, and incisions must understand the sickness before prescribing the cure. We want dialogue, which leads to empowerment. We defy labels that don't even apply to us. I personally don't want to cover my wounds with a "matching skin" bandage, without anyone addressing the fact that we do not all have the same skin colour. We are different, each of us, unique and special. I call on all Women of Colour and Indigenous Women globally to join in this fight. We need to make safe and healthy spaces for ourselves. We need to heal our minds, bodies, hearts, and souls.

For me this anthology is an attack, a waging of a war against the systemic barriers, the silence, the untold stories, and the unheard voices of women. For example, in looking at HIV/AIDS and the impact on Women of Colour and Indigenous Women, the need to break down and identify barriers becomes quite evident. Statistics show that:

> Over two thirds of all the people living with HIV in the world, 25.3 million men, women, and children, live in Sub-Sahara Africa (UNAIDS/WHO). Today, of the estimated 36.1 million people living with HIV/AIDS, an estimated 16.4 million, or 45 percent of all people living with HIV/AIDS are women (UNAIDS/WHO).[3]

Reports have also indicated that in Canada there are high rates of maternal-infant infection with the virus among Caribbean and African Women. In Canada, "between 1994 and 1996, 70 per cent of maternal-infant transmission of HIV infection had occurred among persons from HIV-endemic regions, mainly Africa and the Caribbean."[4] In Canada a large population of African and Caribbean Women are HIV-positive and/or living with AIDS, yet quite a disproportional amount of these women are excluded from research and policy making.[5]

To further illustrate my point, the minimal amount of information and research available reveals that HIV and AIDS rates are increasing at alarming rates within Aboriginal communities, especially among Aboriginal women.[6] The research also shows that infection is occurring in very young Aboriginal women, much younger than in non-Aboriginal women. Yet Aboriginal women have not been the centre or the focus for research on AIDS/HIV prevention or cure. These communities of women remain on the margins with little or no attention being paid to health issues and concerns that are affecting their communities in devastating and tragic ways.[7]

I know that globally women face immense oppressions. I think we can all agree that violence and sickness affects us all. Therefore, let us join forces in combat and do what is needed to stop the pain. Let us focus on prevention, deconstructing the way we define health and establishing systems in our society dedicated to women participating in decisions surrounding their health and well-being; let's move from the notion that health is for the lucky and the wealthy to the realization that health is for all of us. To all women who fight pain daily, for all the tears we hold back, for all the unnecessary deaths and for all the necessary triumphs, this book is a podium, a banner, and a memorandum for you.

Endnotes

1 *Promoting the Health and Well Being of South Asian Women: A Health Promotion Project* (South Asian Community and Region of Peel Health Department, Winter 1999) 13.

2 Carol Amaratunga, ed., *Race, Ethnicity and Women's Health* (Atlantic Centre of Excellence for Women's Health, Nova Scotia, 2002), 187.

3 "Black Women and HIV/AIDS Contextualizing their Realities, their Silence and Proposing Solutions," *Canadian Women Studies* 21, no. 2 (Women and HIV/AIDS issue): 72.

4 Ibid., 73.

5 Ibid., 73.

6 "HIV/AIDS and Aboriginal Women in Canada," *Canadian Women Studies* 21, no. 2 (Women and HIV/AIDS Issue): 25.

7 Ibid., 25.

Perspectives on Health in the Diaspora

UNDERSTANDING THE CHALLENGES

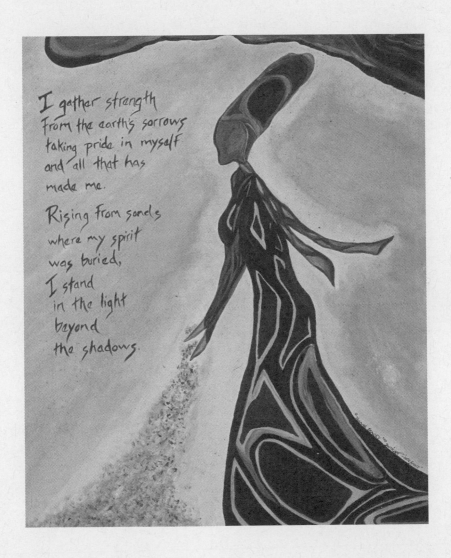

I gather strength
From the earth's sorrows
taking pride in myself
and all that has
made me.

Rising from sands
where my spirit
was buried,
I stand
in the light
beyond
the shadows.

Nurses in Resistance

KAREN FLYNN

My decision to research and write about the experiences of Black
Canadian and Caribbean immigrant nurses has been avowedly
political. The goal is to ensure that the experiences of these women
and their contributions to the political economy of Canada is documented and not lost in historical obscurity. This particular research
is significant in that it validates Black women as producers of knowledge in a society that often ignores and attempts to locate Blacks
generally on the periphery of political and social life. The purpose of
this paper is to examine the multiple resistance strategies employed
by Black nurses working in hospitals where they were either the
only Black or were one of two Black nurses. Because nursing has
historically been defined as a gendered occupation premised on the
ethos of caring, issues of racism and differential treatment are rarely
addressed in a serious way. However, despite the challenges that
Black nurses face – particularly those who immigrated during the
1970s, or entered the occupation in the 1980s when the occupation
was undergoing intense transformation – Black nurses have always
defined themselves as professionals. Beginning with Black Canadian-born and then immigrant nurses who helped to fill the labour
shortage following World War II, these women continue to carve
out a space for themselves in nursing. Therefore, in keeping with the
theme of this anthology, I would like to focus on a few of the resistance strategies Black nurses utilized, to show how these methods
can be used to maintain one's health, well-being, and survival.

In societies where inequalities exist, parents are often credited
with introducing their children to early forms of resistance as ways
to nurture their spirits. As girls, Black Canadian-born nurses knew

from an early age the perniciousness of racism to their daily existence. It is from women such as Edna Black Searles, Laura Tynes, Marlene Watson, and Darlene Barnes that we get a glimpse into how Canada was for Black families. These women discussed a period in Canadian history that mirrored to a certain extent the segregation of the American South; an era that most White Canadians would feign amnesia or deny ever existed. Tynes and Barnes, who grew up in Nova Scotia, spoke about the covert and sometimes subtle racism that Blacks faced daily. They recounted how Blacks were excluded from entering certain public spaces, and the lack of jobs and opportunities available to them. Barnes pointed out that her father prepared her for dealing with racism by making ongoing comparisons to the United States. She remembered:

> He [her father] would talk about Canada as though Canada was no better than the United States, and it wasn't. They had the same 'Whites only' restaurants, Whites only drinking fountains. Blacks were expected to go to the back of the bus. Canada truly wants the world to believe that racism did not exist here; that was an American thing. But guess what, it was blatant as hell in this country.

To protect and prepare their children to deal with the everyday forms of racism faced in their communities, parents were credited with introducing ideas of early resistance. These girls were told to either ignore the derogatory and racist name-calling or, in the case of Barnes, to respond with physical retaliation. According to Barnes, "by the time you smacked the kids, they stopped, they never called you nigger again." Thus parents instilled in their children a sense of pride about being Black – the idea that they were not inferior and were just as good as Whites – as well as emphasizing the significance of education and achievement. Tynes, for example, pointed out that:

> My mother always seemed to find money to buy books and so on to get us doing educational things. [She] was always in the background, attempting to teach us and make ways for us to achieve whatever we wanted to achieve.

The nurses extracted from the crucial lessons of survival learned as children and incorporated these tenets in their adult life.

In *From Stumbling Blocks to Stepping Stones: The Life Experiences of Fifty Professional African American Women*, Kathleen F. Selvin and C. Ray Wingrove point out that for Black girls growing up in a racially divided America a good education was seen as the "passport to a better life." This emphasis on acquiring a formal education is not exclusively a Black American phenomenon, but is applicable to other Black girls living in other parts of the world especially those from poor and working-class backgrounds. This focus on the value of education propounded to Black girls exemplifies resistance especially when looking at how education remained significant throughout the careers of the nurses under discussion. Education was used as a tool by Black nurses as a way of remaining competitive, but also as proof that that they were indeed qualified and skilled professionals in comparison to their White counterparts.

The significance of pursuing education as a way of resisting devaluation in nursing is reflected in the experiences of British-trained Caribbean, and Caribbean-trained nurses who immigrated to Canada due to an acute nursing shortage following World War II. Due to the inability of nursing associations, and later the College of Nurses, to decipher the qualifications and experience of this group of nurses, many were forced to accept positions for which they were overqualified. This process of de-skilling initially affected the self-esteem of these nurses. Accustomed to more autonomy and responsibilities in Britain and the Caribbean, they found themselves in Canada doing what Elaine McCleod classified as "non-educational tasks." Elaborating on her first job at the Toronto Western Hospital, McCleod recalled:

> I wasn't doing a whole lot, and it was frustrating. You were coming from somewhere where you were accustomed to running a whole unit, to do all your orders, and carry out all your assignments that the doctors gave you, and having come here you can't do nothing. You couldn't do dressing, you couldn't give meds. All you could do was make beds, feed, and bathe patients.

Even though the majority of nurses felt that the experience, skills, and training from Britain and the Caribbean prepared them to work in Canada, in order to access and regain those positions they held in Britain, upgrading was essential. Thus, in order to be considered fully-fledged professionals in terms of Canadian standards, these nurses took the required courses and exams.

Coupled with obtaining the necessary education, Caribbean nurses also expressed a profound sense of confidence in their training, skills, and experience, which they felt superseded that of their White Canadian counterparts. Belief in one's ability to *be the best* is an adage that these nurses relied on in order to work within an environment whereupon migration they faced de-skilling, and their training was not always respected and valued. Caribbean British and Caribbean trained nurses knew they exemplified the epitome of professionalism, and repeatedly referred to this in the interviews. Jennette Prince summed up what the majority of these nurses knew about themselves and their abilities. "The assumption was that British trained nurses didn't have the theory, but we got them both together." Prince pointed out that although Canadian nurses might have passed their exams, "they were not good nurses. It was rare to find a good nurse because (a) they were not used to looking after more than two patients, and (b) they were not used to being on their own." Thus, resistance is embodied in rejecting the subordination associated with being de-skilled. While these nurses discussed the frustrations they felt while dealing with the nursing bureaucracy, as well as being located on the bottom of the nursing hierarchy, they often relied on their own knowledge about their abilities to do nursing. In order to cope, these nurses drew on their own notions of professionalism by highlighting and comparing their training and experience to that of Canadian nurses.

In examining power relations in health care, it is accepted that nurses occupy a subordinate position in a male dominated profession.[1] Thus, it is not uncommon for scholars to explore how patriarchy defines and influences that relationship. In focusing on gender, the issue of racism in Canadian nursing has been seriously neglected or downplayed. How Black nurses have experienced and dealt with racism, and the day-to-day realities of nursing, depended on the period in which they immigrated and the extent to which racism was politicized. Furthermore, changes in the structure of the occupation was also a major factor influencing Black nurses' experience. Nurses who came in the 1950s and 1960s pointed out that they did not face much racism, and if an incident occurred that could be construed as racist, it only appeared to have racial overtones in the context of today's society. These early migrants pointed out that they were accepted and treated well because of (1) the nursing shortage, and (2) that racism was tempered because Blacks were few in numbers. Monica Mitchell pointed out that:

> I have often said to people that when I came to Canada the first time, I was comfortable. I never heard all this Black and White thing, and my feeling is that my group did not represent a threat to White people. Now I think my group is a threat.

Vera Cudjoe also expressed similar sentiments:

> The issue of racism was not evident and apparent at that time as it is now. There were so few of us here they had (meaning Whites) not begin to panic, to feel afraid, or intimidated by our presence…. On the other hand, in the hospital we were a minority and we were just concerned about doing our work. They seemed to want us more than anything else.

The earlier migrants did discuss racism outside of nursing, particularly in terms of housing. Within nursing it was difficult to assess situations as racist, and thus many nurses found other plausible explanations for their victimization. In thinking about whether she had ever experienced racism, Cudjoe pointed out:

> I was not aware of racism at that time about racism, but in hindsight I think there was, because there were times when

people were being unfair and you didn't know why. You never thought it was because of me being Black. You were more concerned with the actual victimization of what's being done to you and trying to work it out and resolve it, rather than point at somebody else and call them a racist.

In many ways, the nurses' refusal to see or discuss racism within nursing can be seen as another form of resistance. In so doing, racist and sexual oppression did not emerge as the only factor determining the nurses' existence.

That racism did not emanate as the primary explanation for how Black nurses were treated, allowed them to perform their tasks without the stress associated with believing that racism permeates every aspect of nursing. Thus, as Cudjoe pointed out, "We were just concerned with doing our work." For these women, nursing was viewed as a type of calling, a way of helping others, and despite the racism or other inequalities that might have existed in the workplace, these nurses were fulfilling a dream, and they were often mindful of this reality when working.

Another form of resistance is being cognizant of limits, which is illustrated in the number of nurses who frequently changed jobs because of incidents with White nurses or administrators. For example, Lillie Johnson was placed on a difficult floor and left the job because she believed that being on that floor would preclude moving up the nursing hierarchy. As stated before, these nurses did not always construe these incidents as being racist, but rather characterized tensions in terms of personality differences, education, or experience. One nurse maintained that she only spent three weeks at a hospital and left after being bossed around by a less-qualified White nurse. Likewise, Johnson's tenure at the St. Joseph's hospital was also brief because, as she recalled, "It was the most difficult floor. Anytime there is a difficult floor that is where they would push Black people." Johnson had aspirations in terms of her career, and left for the Hospital for Sick Children, which provided the support needed to obtain her registration. While formal acts of resistance would involve, for example, registering complaints with the appropriate bodies in nursing, these nurses did not choose this avenue; which does not make their choice of frequent hospital moves, in terms of thinking about resistance, any less valid.

At the same time, dealing with all the issues surrounding being migrants in a new country was also very daunting. As a result, resistance can also be identified in the methods adopted by the earlier immigrants. Because they were so few Blacks in Canada generally, in order to make the transition of being immigrants smoother, nurses such as Mitchell interacted with other immigrants who were in a similar predicament of being new to the society. Thus, for example, they socialized at the YWCA who organized dances for immigrants. Cudjoe explained a typical Friday night at the YWCA:

> On Friday nights we would attend the YWCA; it was very multicultural, they catered to everyone. I met a lot of men of men from Europe. They came from Europe to work. They were Germans, Hungarians, and Italians. We dated some of these people and some of my friends got married to some of these people.

The early immigrant nurses also befriended nurses from other cultural backgrounds, as well as White Canadian nurses. In the interviews, it is not uncommon for nurses to say, "we are still friends up until today." These nurses are proud of their ability to interact and develop friendships with people that were not necessarily from their country of origin, because it represented their ability to adapt to a new society.

Nurses who immigrated reflected in the latter decades when racism was more politicized, and developed their own methods of dealing and coping with the differential treatment they faced. Having seen their counterparts fired, offered packages because of cutbacks in health care, or demoted, some nurses preferred to ignore racism than deal with the consequences of speaking out. In her contemporary study on racism in nursing, Tania Das Gupta points out, that "targeting outspoken nurses of colour seems to be a common experience. Typically, a Black nurse is singled out and subjected to differential treatment by management compared to White workers."[2] Dorothy Jones, for example, remembered one such nurse in particular who stood out in her mind. According to Jones, this nurse would:

> ... stand up for her rights. She was able to stand up to them and fight for her rights. She would go to whoever she to go to to get her satisfaction; and so [she] was branded a trouble-maker. But it's because she was able to stand up to them (meaning Whites) and they didn't like this girl at all. She didn't care. If she had to take it to the union or whatever to fix whatever was wrong, she did it.

Those nurses who often took the chance of speaking out without fear of being penalized did so because for them it was a question of integrity. Others, such as Verna Barrett, who faced racism from a doctor, who had four other Black nurses fired, relied on more formal mechanisms such as the union. She recalled:

> I phoned the union, and they showed up.... This doctor's name apparently rang a bell, and I told him what happened. He told them, he said "we're willing to go to court, if there isn't an apology." So I got my apology.

Some nurses accepted that racism in nursing was inevitable and did not let its impact on their lives affect their ability to perform their work, or their mental health. Making a decision to remain silent in the face of oppression should not be construed as a sign of weakness, but as another form of resistance, *choosing one's battles carefully*. When Black nurses experienced indignation or rage at particular injustices, they often relied on their friends and colleagues to listen and validate their experiences. Patricia Hill Collins reminds us that:

> ... while domination may be an inevitable social fact, it is unlikely to be hegemonic ideology within that social

space where Black women can speak freely. This realm of relatively safe discourse, however narrow, is a necessary condition for Black women's resistance.[3]

Black nurses relied on public spaces, such as their churches, cultural organizations, as well friendships they formed primarily with other Black nurses to talk about the inequalities they faced. Elaine McLeod described her relationship with the women she worked with upon migration from Britain in the following way: "I could relate to them more, and they had a bit of understanding from where you were coming from, and what you were able to do, having to work here [Canada]." Sandra Ward described working with her "own people," as being healthy and worthwhile. She pointed out, "It's been good, we can talk with each other rather than with other people." The multiple experiences these nurses faced were then validated and legitimized in the confines of formal organizations or among friends.

Resistance also comes in the form of *lifting as you climb*. Many Black nurses discussed how fruitful it was to assist other nurses and be assisted by other nurses to *learn the ropes*. Black nurses often encouraged their sisters to advance their education. One nurse pointed out that:

> if the health care aid doesn't know something we help them. We have encouraged a lot of them. We'll tell them "you are doing a great job, why don't you do the RPN (Registered Practical Nursing) program and from there you can go further."

Although there were differences in terms of training, experience, and pay, being Black women served to homogenize these women. Thus they overlooked or downplayed their differences in order to *get along* and support each other. Likewise, Lilli Johnson discussed how she saw her role as an older more experienced nurse in relation to younger Black nurses who were experiencing difficulties in the occupation. Johnson maintained, "I wanted to elevate and improve their self-esteem, because if you didn't feel good about yourself being Black, you are not going anywhere." For Black nurses the importance of assisting other Black nurses could be characterized as *uplifting the race.* These women had a keen sense of responsibility towards their fellow nurses, especially those concentrated in the lower ranks in the occupation.

Because this involved formal methods of resistance, the various forms of resistance employed by these nurses may not, by scholarly standards, be defined as such, but they are indeed significant because they worked. Black nurses, whether from the Caribbean or Canada, faced similar struggles associated with having Black skin, as well as the additional struggles associated with being nurses. These women adopted multiple forms of resistance to deal with the reality of working in Canadian hospitals and civil society. These forms of resistance can also be utilized by Black and women of colour who are interested in having a stake in their own well-being, as they struggle daily against racist-sexist inequalities and other forms of oppression endemic in this society.

Endnotes

1   See, for example, Pat Armstrong, Jacqueline Choiniere, and Elaine Day, *Vital signs: Nursing in transition* (Garamond Press, 1993). Barbara Keddy et al., Nurses' work world: Scientific or womanly ministering. *Resources for Feminist Research,* 7(3): 99–102; Kathryn McPherson, *Bedside matters: The transformation of Canadian nursing, 1900–1990* (Toronto: Oxford University Press, 1996).
2   Tania Das Gupta, *Racism and paid work.* (Garamond Press: 1996), 75.
3   Patricia Hill Collins, *Black feminist thought: Knowledge, consciousness and the politics of empowerment* (London: Routledge, 1991), 94.

African-Canadian Women Resisting Oppression: Embodying Emancipated Consciousness through Holistic Self-Healing Approaches to Mental Health

DR. INGRID R.G. WALDRON, PH.D.

Racism as a Mental Health Issue

Racism is the most important mental health issue affecting the lives of people of colour. It produces the psycho-social stressors that lead to mental health problems and is a major barrier to access or utilization of mental health services. The fact that racial abuse has yet to be recognized in the DSM (American Psychiatric Association Diagnostic and Statistical Manual of Mental Disorder) as a valid mental health problem, may have much to do with a tendency in North America to undermine or ignore the significant impact of racism on mental health.

This paper identifies how oppressive structures, processes, and relations produce the various psycho-social stressors that impact on the mental health of African-Canadian women. It also inquires into the psychological impact of racial abuse on African-Canadian women. I expand the Euro-Western notion of pathology and *mental illness* as being rooted in some biological and genetic malfunctioning, to the notion of these concepts as being produced from the psychological violence, spiritual, and psychic abuse and annihilation that are perpetrated against racialized peoples in Euro-Western societies.

I was born in Montreal, Quebec to middle-class Trinidadian parents who had immigrated to Montreal to pursue university studies. As a child growing up in Canada, I experienced racism in its most overt and abusive forms as a victim of racial slurs and physical harassment and violence. And, although I was too young to understand it at the time, racial divisions in this country had constructed me as *undesirable, the other,* and an outsider who did not belong. Moreover, although I have always resented being made to feel like an outsider by some White people (many of whom are themselves immigrants) solely because of my race, I appreciate that it is impossible for me to identify with the *immigrant experience* in this country. Despite the fact that I share similar experiences of racial discrimination with many Black immigrant groups, I simultaneously occupy a privileged position in relation to those whose immigrant status serves to bar them from accessing various institutional resources.

When I emigrated to Trinidad with my family in the late 1970s, I experienced a shift in my identity from being a person who was a member of a racially subordinated group to a person who was now a member of the dominant group numerically, culturally, racially, and politically. In Trinidad, race was no longer salient for me. I was no longer *Black, a person of colour,* or *a visible minority.* And, although my *Canadianness* (dress, accent, culture, values) was a source of interest and curiosity for the other students, I was never *treated* as an outsider who did not belong. Unlike in Canada, where *the immigrant* is a socially constructed concept designed to exclude and oppress those members of society perceived to be undesirable because of nationality, culture, ethnicity, race, language, and religion, the concept holds no such currency in Trinidad.

What did become salient for me in Trinidad was my status as a member of a privileged class in a society where a rigid stratification system based on class has endured since slavery. Before I emigrated to Trinidad, I never had to consider how my father's status as a dentist provided me with certain material and non-material privileges. It was only when I moved to Trinidad did I come to understand (usually prompted by outspoken students who took it upon themselves to constantly remind me of this fact) how his socio-economic status in a country with a substantial working-class population accorded me certain benefits and rewards that were denied to others.

When I returned to Canada five years later, I did so armed with a perspective that had been transformed substantially. Not only had I grown accustomed to (and grown to love) my life in a Black-dominated society, but I had also begun to experience my racial identity in a novel way. Although I had already experienced overt forms of racism (physical harassment, verbal abuse) as a child growing up in Canada, I was now able to identify the more sophisticated, covert, subtle, and emotionally damaging form of racism that operated within various institutions such as employment. I came to understand how I had to work twice as hard and be twice as good in a workplace where I was more educationally qualified than many of my White peers. I also recognized how my failure to secure various work promotions that I was clearly and undisputedly qualified for in this White female-dominated workplace had everything to do with my membership in a racially excluded group that continues to be confronted with the perennial *glass ceiling*.

It is these experiences that have had the most damaging impact on me and many Black people emotionally and psychologically, resulting in our frustration, anger, and, at times, doubt that we will be allowed to realize our full potential in the same way that many of our White counterparts will. When racialized peoples are constrained by the limitations imposed by a racially stratified society, hopelessness, helplessness, frustration, and anger will inevitably result. So, it truly mystifies me when White people fail to comprehend the anger and frustrations of Black people in this society. When White people dismiss *Black anger* as a mere childish *knee-jerk* response to not getting what we want, how and when we want it, they not only imply that racism is not a real phenomenon operating in the lives of racialized peoples, but they also fail to appreciate the debilitating and damaging psychological impact of racism, as well as its role in producing various mental health problems, such as depression, stress, and addictions. Instead, when racialized peoples express the pain and hurt of racism, they are often accused of over-reacting, and of being too emotional, sensitive, paranoid, suspicious, and irrational.

Schreiber, Noerager, and Wilson (1998, p. 511) found that there are an estimated 200,000 Black women in Canada, with the vast majority having immigrated from the Caribbean. She also found that there are approximately 44,000 adult women who identify themselves as Black in metropolitan Toronto. The increase in immigration numbers and the large numbers of African-Canadian women demand that the mental health system begin to respond to their needs by developing policies and practices that are not only culturally sensitive but that also challenge the race, gender, and class oppression that are interlocked for African-Canadian women and other women of colour. The following section identifies some of the more prevalent institutional structures that may produce mental health problems among African-Canadian people and other minoritized populations.

Identifying the Structures and Processes of Oppression

African-Canadian women and other Black women are subjected to multiple oppressions because of their race, culture, gender, class, and sexual orientation. It is impossible to separate or disentangle these constructs when discussing both their simultaneous enmeshment within the structures and processes of domination and their involvement in producing and exacerbating mental health problems among these women. Perhaps the two most prevalent institutional and social practices that impact on Black women's mental health can be found within the sites of health and employment.

Barbee and Little (1993, p. 182) concluded that the "multiple jeopardies" that result from racism, sexism, poverty, and heterosexism interact in ways that subject Black women worldwide to inadequate housing, limited access to health care facilities, inadequate nutrition, and poor environmental sanitation. These factors expose Black women to multiple health hazards, compromise their health status, and result in lower life expectancy among Black women than White women. For poor African-American women, the ability to resolve their health concerns is affected by their inability to pay for insurance and hospital entrance fees which, in turn, greatly affects their ability to access health services.

The literature also suggests that health statistics are used as instruments of oppression when they demonstrate that African-

Americans suffer disproportionately from specific illnesses and diseases but are, instead, used to ameliorate the health problems of White members of the population. Consequently, the health of African-American people is put at risk when the health system determines them ineligible for treatment based on inequitable practices that undermine their health concerns. Barbee and Little (1993) found that, despite the fact that statistics have long showed that African-American women suffer disproportionately from such serious illnesses as hypertension, malnutrition, psycho-social deprivation, lupus, diabetes, maternal mortality, and cervical cancer, the health care sector has largely continued to turn a blind eye to this fact, focusing instead on the health concerns of White Americans.

A study conducted by the Ministry of Health of Ontario (1993) looked at the health care experiences of minority women in Ontario and found that these women are discriminated against by the Ontario health care system because of racism, limited language and literacy levels, and lack of economic opportunities. The study found that racially differentiated women are perceived to be inferior by White Canadian health care providers and that they confront various structural barriers, including lack of access to language training and ghettoization in low paying jobs, both of which restrict their opportunities to access health services.

Several studies have also found that African-Canadian people suffer disproportionately from discriminatory practices in employment. Carey (2001) found that inequitable practices in employment in Toronto confine many new immigrants of colour to job ghettos that are characterized by low pay, menial tasks, and poor working conditions. Similarly, Ornstein (2000) found that in Toronto the most severe disadvantage affects African ethno-racial groups, such as Ethiopians, Ghanaians, Somalis, and other African nations. These groups suffer high rates of poverty, which reflect their high levels of unemployment and concentration in low-skill employment. Only Afghans live in comparably difficult circumstances. A number of African, Black, and Caribbean ethno-racial groups experience more poverty than any other ethno-racial group in Toronto and have family incomes below the Toronto average.

Ornstein's report (2000) found that almost half of all Somali men and women are in lower skill manual occupations and that more than 80 per cent of Ethiopian women and 70 per cent of Ethiopian men are in lower skill manual or non-manual occupations. He also found that Black women from Africa and the Caribbean are especially disadvantaged in relation to Black men from these countries, with a median income of $25,000 compared to $26,000 for Black men, $30,000 for other female ethno-racial groups, and $35,000 for other male ethno-racial groups. This data suggests that these women encounter high levels of injustice, discrimination, and oppression within dominant structures which, in turn, may impact significantly on their psychological well-being. It is critical then, that researchers and practitioners begin to unmask the racial, gender, and class inequalities that run rampant in the structures and processes of domination in Canada and to critically question how those social oppressors converge to produce the psycho-social stressors that lead to mental health problems among African-Canadian women.

Brand (1999) and Sharma (1994) found that visible minorities in Canada, for the most part, have been forced to take the jobs that the White population does not want in the low wage, labour-intensive, and underdeveloped sectors. Sharma found that women of colour earned 51 per cent of what White men earned and 59 per cent of what men of colour earned. Brand concluded that eight out of ten Black people in Canada have family members who are employed in service work as domestics, factory labourers, nursing assistants and attendants, hotel cleaners, and maids.

Elabor-Idemudia (2000, p. 91) found that immigrant and refugee women from the Caribbean and Africa tend to come to Canada as family members under the family reunification program with high-level skills and education. Despite this, many of them encounter discrimination when they attempt to access employment and are barred from the processes and structures that facilitate social mobility and assimilation into Canadian society. Women who enter as independent-class immigrants with high level education and skills are often forced to accept the low status jobs that tend to be reserved for Black women and other women of colour. These jobs are characterized by low wages, part-time hours, low job security, and occupational and industrial segregation. Elabor-Idemudia (p. 91) also found that immigration and citizenship laws are most oppressive to racialized women because of patriarchal, racist, and sexist ideologies that require sponsored immigrant women to depend on the goodwill of a male principal applicant's approval of the sponsorship agreement.

In my study (Waldron, 2002), I found that one of the more damaging characteristics of Euro-Western institutions is how they are able to mask oppression by redefining racism, sexism, and other forms of injustice in ways that make them appear natural and normal. When oppression is normalized in this way, it undermines the existence and experience of racism, sexism, and other oppressions, and ignores or negates the impact of these oppressions on victims. Moreover, the responsibility to identify and prove racism may often be placed on the victim. As a result, oppressed peoples will often internalize racism and other social oppressions when they are unable to identify or admit to how these oppressions constrict and restrict their lives, and when they are made to feel that the injustices they suffer are the result of their own perceived shortcomings.

In my study I interviewed eleven informants. Six of these informants were African-Canadian mental health professionals, four were African-Canadian women who had been diagnosed with mental health problems and are receiving treatment, and one was an African-Canadian female who had never accessed a mental health site but had received support from friends. Although this informant had never accessed a mental health site, I felt that her account of how racism had impacted upon her emotional well-being was a crucial component of my study.

My study (Waldron, 2002) identified the most common psychosocial stressors for African Canadian women (apart from or because of racism) as being (a) poor education, (b) poor health, (c) employment discrimination, (d) unemployment and underemployment, (e) single parent/motherhood, (f) poverty, (g) housing discrimination, (h) poor nutrition, (i) family dislocation, and (j) migration. The feelings of discrimination experienced by my informants contributed significantly to the severe mental health problems that many of them suffer from today.

For many of the informants in my study, employment discrimination has been the prime contributor to the mental health problems that they struggle with today. Some of the women in my study told of how they have had to confront the glass ceiling in their workplaces when they were denied promotional opportunities or were not nurtured by management to take advantage of certain employment opportunities. There was also a general sentiment among my informants that African-Canadian people are set up to fail in this country. In the following section, I discuss the impact of oppression on mental health.

The Psychology of Oppression

Black peoples who live in Euro-Western societies are often victims of consistent and persistent ideological indoctrination from Euro-Western society, media, and educational institutions. The negative outcomes for these peoples are alienation, disaffection, and oppression due to cultural, political, social, academic, and economic underachievement, as well as mental, psychological, and spiritual destitution.

Although cultural influences on the conceptualizations of *mental illness* and help-seeking have been considerably investigated in the research, fewer researchers have sought to examine the significance of racism in the discourse and practice of psychiatry and in the production of psycho-social stressors that lead to mental health problems. The authors who have endeavoured to do this (Across Boundaries, 1997; Azibo, 1989; Baldwin, 1980; Canadian Task Force on Mental Health Issues Affecting Immigrants and Refugees, 1988; Fanon, 1963; Fernando, 1988; Jenkins, 1995; Nobles, 1976; Wright, 1974) documented the devastating impact of oppression on the mental health of Black people and people of colour.

Fanon (1963) stated that the abuse that colonial domination and oppression inflicts on the colonized personality results in a profound sensitivity, the erosion of self-respect and self-worth, and, consequently, mental pathology. He argued (1963, p. 249) that it was inevitable that colonialism would prove fertile ground for the production of psychiatric and behavioural problems among the colonized. Fanon was less concerned with the superficial particularities of racial stereotypes that were at the centre of Eurocentric discourse than with the exploitation of racial difference for economic and political gain.

Fernando (1998, p. 227) also argued that racism represents a psychological assault on the sense of self and that the devaluation and demoralization that Black people experience as a result of racism leaves them spiritually destitute, disconnected, and alienated. Similarly, Jenkins (1995, p. 228) argued that Black people suffer a kind of "cultural depression" because they are victims of racist practices that limit their social opportunities, making it difficult for them to establish strong interpersonal relationships, families, and community organizations. He also stated that although this *cultural depression* may not show up in clinical depression, it is more pervasive.

Baldwin (1980, p. 100) expounded on this notion of "racism as violence" by arguing that Europeans are able to gain psychological control over non-European peoples by imposing a Eurocentric worldview upon them. He (1984, p. 179) blamed the weakening and distortion of the Black personality on the imposition of an alien or non-African influence on African-American people. He saw the socio-cultural and mental health problems of African-Americans as being the result of the unnatural influence of a Western and Eurocentric cosmology that is substantially at odds with an African cosmology. Baldwin also argued (p. 184) that African-Americans have adopted a false sense of consciousness as a result of being socialized and indoctrinated by an alien influence that is Eurocentric and anti-African. This influence, he concedes, produces negative self-concepts in African-Americans that result in destructive behaviours and that, consequently, threaten the survival of the group.

Wright (1974) coined the term "mentacide" to refer to the "silent rape" of a people's collective mind by the penetration and perpetuation of alien culture, values, belief systems, or ideas for the purpose of group destruction. He argued that mentacide occurs when subordinate groups accept and internalize the culture, values, and belief systems of the dominant group. It damages African self-consciousness, causing African peoples of the diaspora to adopt the behavioural characteristics of the oppressor. Similarly, Azibo (1989, p. 186) used the term "alienating mentacide" to refer to the process of indoctrination that commands acceptance of and respect for a Euro-centric value system and promotes negative depictions of African peoples.

According to a study conducted by Across Boundaries (1997, p. 5), people of colour and First Nations people in Canada who live in restrictive environments face oppressive circumstances that put them at increased risk for drug and alcohol addiction, violent crimes, and stress and stress-related illnesses. The Canadian Task Force on Mental Health Issues Affecting Immigrants and Refugees (1988) described the impact of discrimination in Canada on mental health in this way:

> The basis for much of the mental health problems in Canada is moderate, systemic racism throughout our society.... The racism that lingers is still powerful enough to place visible minority people under the pressure of always being on watch for the hard edge of prejudice and discrimination. It is the individual representations of this racist plague that underlies, we think, many of the psycho-social problems immigrants and refugees manifest (p. 12).

These works were crucial to my study (Waldron, 2002) because they provided me with a framework with which to articulate how oppressive circumstances impact on the mental, psychological, emotional, and spiritual well-being of African-Canadian women. Their conceptualization of racism as abusive and violent is one that I rely on in my work, mainly because of the failure of the DSM and other psychological and psychiatric literature to define it in this way. I was interested in looking at how the broader, micro-political structures of the colonial encounter (i.e., Euro-Western societies) impinge on the mental health of Black women. I also look at the actions that these women engage in to subvert and challenge dominant structures and processes.

My understanding of pathology moves beyond the traditional Western psychiatric conceptualization of it as having a biological and genetic basis to an understanding of it as being the culmination of consistent and persistent racial abuse and indoctrination into an alien culture. In this way, my study uses the *colonial pathologies* concept to refer to those mental health problems that are produced from living in oppressive societies. These mental health problems are experienced by non-European and racialized peoples who suffer from feelings of subordination, subjugation, and oppression within colonial relations and imperial structures in these societies.

Several of the mental health professionals in my research saw an urgent need for the DSM, and the psychiatric profession as a whole, to articulate *mental illness* within the context of the macro-political structures of society, and to acknowledge how people's experiences are filtered through race and other social oppressions. They cited as problematic the DSM's failure to acknowledge racism as a mental health issue in terms of its involvement in the production of the psycho-social stressors that impact on the mental, emotional, psychological, and spiritual well-being of racialized peoples.

Several of the mental health professionals in my study argued that it was important for the psychiatric profession to make distinctions between *mental illness* (psychiatric disorder) and the mental health problems that are produced by psycho-social stressors when discussing African-Canadian women. They argued that the needs of individuals will differ depending on whether they are suffering from the *mental illnesses* that have their origins in an internal source (i.e., biological, chemical) or an external one (i.e., psycho-social stressors). There was a general sentiment that while the use of scientific constructs may be appropriate in many cases to understand, explain, and treat *mental illness* within mental health sites, treatment for psycho-social problems should involve helping the patient identify and eradicate all the determinants of mental health problems, including such day-to-day concerns as housing, employment, literacy, immigration and refugee issues, and child care.

My study identified Black refugees and Black immigrants in Canada as being most at risk for experiencing the psycho-social stressors that may lead to mental health problems because, in addition to coping with racism, sexism, and poverty, they must also deal with the hopelessness, helplessness, and anguish that is often the result of having unfulfilled expectations in a new country. Similarly, in a recent study (Gajardo and Waldron, 2001) on the experiences of refugee students in higher education institutions in Canada, it was found that the social and emotional well-being of refugees is hampered by such pre-migration situations as persecution, famine, state violence, and detention camps, which, in turn impact on the ways in which these groups cope with cultural dislocation, precarious residency status, family breakdown, isolation, unemployment, underemployment, and legal problems. These factors are further compounded by discriminatory and racist processes within Canadian institutions that are designed to deny refugees access to social, economic, and educational opportunities in Canada.

My study (Waldron, 2002) suggests that African-Canadian women who must deal with limited social opportunities often experience a kind of *spiritual impotence* that results in a sense of powerlessness, helplessness, hopelessness, and worthlessness, and that forces them to respond with rage, anger, sadness, apathy, and anxiety. By spiritual impotence, I mean the feeling of being incapacitated and castrated emotionally by oppressive structures that inhibit these women from realizing their full potential. In essence, these women's hopes, dreams, and desires are curtailed severely by discriminatory practices and processes that deter them from achieving spiritual fulfilment. What was most commonly articulated in my study was how experiences of oppression contributed to these women's low self-esteem, depression, stress, intellectual and mental deterioration (like memory loss, in the case of one of my informants), and addictions. Several of the informants argued that racism had killed their spirit, eroding the core of who they were as individuals and leaving them without the necessary coping mechanisms and will to actively engage in their lives.

My study was also particularly concerned with demonstrating how African-Canadian women can use an understanding of the self, their environment, and, most importantly, their culture and history to develop self-healing approaches that offer a counter stance to the imposing, dominating, and, often, denigrating knowledge in psychiatry. For African peoples of the diaspora, liberation or what I refer to as "emancipated consciousness" is embodied in liberation from ideological, mental, and psychological dominance and in the capacity to construct self-valuations that subvert normative assumptions about Black people, Black history, and Black culture in Euro-Western societies.

In the following section, I elaborate on how an emancipated consciousness for my informants is embodied in self-healing approaches that subvert and transform dominant conceptions of *mental illness*. I demonstrate how women who have been psychologically impacted by experiences of oppression can become more empowered by engaging in self-healing approaches that combine the indigenous healing practices of their ancestors with Western psychiatric approaches.

Emancipated Consciousness through Self-Healing

Pajaczkowska and Young (1992, p. 198) state that the psychoanalytic emphasis on the complex and often painful transactions between the psychic and social can reveal how deeply racism permeates not only the institutions of post-colonial societies, but also the ways in which we experience ourselves and others. Perhaps the most significant aspect of my research is my examination of how African-Canadian women recover their sense of identity in societies where they are subjected to experiences of intense trauma and dehumanization. I refer to this as "emancipated consciousness" because it describes how the inner workings of Black women's consciousness is shaped by their understandings of the self and their spiritual, psychological, and physical worlds.

Emancipated consciousness also refers to the emotional, mental, spiritual, and psychological liberation that these women attain when they subvert and transform dominant mental health knowledge within marginalized spaces, such as psychiatry. It describes how African-Canadian women resist the marginalization, suppression, and devaluation of their knowledge by interrogating the effectiveness of Euro-Western psychiatry and by reclaiming the mental health knowledge that emanate from their own cultural frames of reference. The African-Canadian women in my study were often involved in a process where they questioned the appropriateness of Euro-Western psychiatric knowledge for their spiritual, emotional, mental, and psychological well-being, and made decisions about when that knowledge should be discarded or retained in the self-healing approaches that they engaged in.

My study found that many African-Canadian women maximize their care by making use of self-healing approaches that combine indigenous healing approaches that emanate from traditional African culture and Euro-Western psychiatric interventions. I found that when the African-Canadian women in my study seek out assistance, they do so by either receiving treatment from formal/professional resources like family doctors, psychiatrists, hospital emergency wards, counselling, and psychotherapy, or from more informal (and non-psychiatric) resources like social support networks of friends and family, church and other religious and spiritual activities, meditation and relaxation, solitude, and diet regulation. Of these approaches, the most common sources of assistance used by these women are social support networks of friends and family and family doctors, and the least used are counselling and therapy.

Many of these women often don't realize that the self-healing approaches they use that combine psychiatry, counselling, therapy, a family doctor, meditation, yoga, solitude, diet regulation, relaxation, social support networks, and religion and spirituality are valid, legitimate, and authentic forms of treatment. This may be because many of these methods take place outside of the confines of formal mental health settings, and, consequently, are not defined by the scientific terminologies and labels of psychiatry.

In essence, then, self-healing characterizes the full range of approaches that these women use to cope with, resolve, and heal their mental health problems, and appropriately describes the creative, diverse, inclusive, and holistic strategies that these women engage in to bring about their own mental, psychological, emotional, spiritual, and physical health. Self-healing can be empowering and liberating because it gives these women a sense of authority over the management of their own health care, requiring that they become autonomous, independent, and, most importantly, active agents in their own health care. It also allows them to use their spiritual, emotional, and intuitive knowledge to monitor, regulate, and respond to their physical, emotional, and spiritual needs on a daily basis. This usually meant constructing individualized self-healing strategies by retaining those approaches that they felt would be most effective and beneficial, and discarding those that would not. My informants' engagement in self-healing was reflective of a shared heritage of oppression and a need to craft a culture of resistance that is informed by individual and collective definitions of Black womanhood. What remained constant was these women's reliance on spirituality as an integral aspect of healing, empowerment, and liberation from oppressive circumstances.

Although the role of spirituality in helping people cope with and resolve mental health problems tends to be downplayed in the psychiatric literature in the West, I found that spirituality and religious activity were crucial in helping some of the women in my study resolve their concerns. Spirituality requires that these women become active participants in their own healing since it often involves independent prayer and a reliance on an inner spiritual strength. The belief in a higher power for dealing with life's hardships has long been an important source of strength for Black people and Black women, in particular. Several authors (Baer, 1981; Boyd-Franklin, 1991; Brown and Gary, 1994; Handel, Black-Lopez and Moergan, 1989; Paris, 1995; The Princeton Religion Research Center, 1987; Schreiber, Noerager, and Wilson, 1998; Stolley and Koenig, 1997; Taylor and Chatters, 1988;) found that religion, spirituality, and the church play a significant role in offsetting the stresses and anxieties that may lead to depression and suicide among African peoples of the diaspora.

Baer (1981) and Paris (1995) both argued that the common belief in a transcendent, divine, and almighty power has been one of the most important components to the continuity between continental Africans and those of the diaspora. Baer (p. 148) found that the belief that one's problems will be solved by establishing a relationship with God is common among peoples of African descent in Africa, the Caribbean, and the United States. Paris (p. 33) stated that African styles of worship, forms of ritual, systems of belief, and fundamental perspectives have been preserved and revitalized on this side of the Atlantic and provide strong evidence that the structural dimensions of African spirituality have been retained.

The Princeton Religion Research Center (1987) found that women, the less educated, and those of lower social classes have been consistently associated with greater religious activity. Taylor and Chatters (1988) found that church members provide a substantial amount of support to many older African-Americans. Stolley and Koenig (1997, p. 34) concluded that religion and spirituality are important sources of support for African-Americans and, similarly, Brown and Gary (1994) found that African-Americans who are active in the church experience fewer depressive symptoms. Handel, Black-Lopez, and Moergan (1989) concluded that Black women who do not participate in religious activities have higher levels of psychological distress than those who do. Boyd-Franklin (1991, p. 37) also stated that spirituality provides a major psychological coping or survival mechanism for many African-American women who experience psychological conflict due to issues of their own sexuality and morality.

Schreiber, Noerager, and Wilson (1998, p. 515) found that African-Canadian women depended quite heavily on God. All of the women in this study were brought up in the church, believed in God, and attended church at least some of the time. They also found that African-Canadian women varied in their belief in Christian doctrine. At one end of the continuum were women who *gave their troubles over* to God, seeking solace and comfort in prayer. At the other end of the continuum were those women who believed in a

God who gave them strength and faith to do what they needed to do in order to resolve their problems. They all prayed routinely, read the Bible, and spoke with God about their pain. For all of the women in this study, religious contemplation provided a diversion and enabled them to direct their thoughts in a more positive direction.

Self-healing enabled my informants to engage in an ongoing process to recover and reclaim their identities by reaching beyond the confines of their concrete, physical environments to the knowledge and practices of their ancestors that were often restricted to intuitive, spiritual, and subjective spaces. They were also able to redefine those spaces by simultaneously rupturing the normative frameworks within which psychiatry operates and by reconfiguring their beliefs, knowledge, and practices within the ideological, intellectual, and physical spaces of the dominant culture. When African-Canadian women situate themselves within these spaces, they achieve an emancipated consciousness because they reconfigure their locations as subordinated and marginalized peoples by engaging in processes of self-empowerment in which they become active agents in developing and legitimizing representations of self and identity. An emancipated consciousness for African-Canadian women, then, is one that strives for higher levels of understanding that are shaped by individual and collective definitions of this group, are grounded in a desire to be free of the material and ideological conditions of oppression and, are embodied in a quest for spiritual, emotional, mental, and psychological liberation.

References

Across Boundaries. (1997). *A guide to anti-racism organizational change in the health and mental health sector.* Toronto: Across Boundaries.

Azibo, D. A. Y. (1989). African-centred theses on mental health and a nosology of Black/African personality disorder. *Journal of Black Psychology 15*(2), 173–214.

Baer, H. (1981). Prophets and advisors in Black spiritual churches: Therapy, palliative or opiate? *Culture, Medicine and Psychiatry 5*, 145–70.

Baldwin, J. A. (1980). The Psychology of oppression. In M. K. Asante, and A. S. Vandi, eds. *Contemporary Black thought: Alternative analyses in social and behavioural science* (pp. 95–110). London: Sage.

Barbee, E. L., and Little, M. (1993). Health, social class and African American women. In S. M. James, and A. P. A. Busia, eds. *Theorizing Black feminisms: The visionary pragmatism of Black women* (pp. 182–99). London: Routledge.

Boyd-Franklin, N. (1991). Recurrent themes in the treatment of African American women in group psychotherapy. *Women and Therapy 11*(2), 25–40.

Brand, D. (1999). Black women and work: The impact of racially constructed gender roles on the sexual division of labour. In E. Dua and A. Robertson, eds. *Scratching the surface: Canadian anti-racist feminist thought* (pp. 83–96). Toronto: Women's Press.

Brown, D. R., and Gary, L. E. (1994). Religious involvement and health status among African American males. *Journal of the National Medical Association 86*, 825–31.

Canadian Task Force on Mental Health Issues Affecting Immigrants and Refugees. (1988). *After the door has opened: Mental health issues affecting immigrants and refugees in Canada.* Ottawa: Minister of Supply and Services Canada.

Carey, E. (2001). The great divide in Toronto housing. *The Toronto Star*, 3 February 2001, pp. M1–M2.

Elabor-Idemudia, P. (2000). Challenges confronting African immigrant women in the Canadian workforce. In A. Calliste and G. J. S. Dei, eds. *Anti-Racist feminism: Critical race and gender studies* (pp. 91–110). Halifax, N.S.: Fernwood.

Fanon, F. (1963). *The wretched of the earth.* New York: Grove Press.

Fernando, S. (1988). *Race and culture in psychiatry.* London: Croom Helm.

Gajardo, L. M., and Waldron, I. R. G. (2000). *A preliminary study evaluating the barriers to greater participation and inclusion of minority students from refugee backgrounds in higher education institutions.* Toronto: University of Toronto, Centre for Integrative Anti-racism Studies.

Handel, P. J., Black-Lopez, W., and Moergan, S. (1989). Preliminary investigation of the relationship between religion and psychological distress in Black women. *Psychological Reports 65*, 971–75.

Jenkins, A. H. (1995). *Psychiatry and African Americans: A humanistic approach*, 2nd ed. Boston: Allyn and Bacon.

Nobles, W. W. (1976). Black people in White insanity: An issue for Black community mental health. *Journal of Afro-American Issues* 4(1), 21–27.

Ministry of Health, Women's Health Bureau. (1993), August. *Immigrant, refugee, and racial minority women and health care needs: A report of community consultations*, no. 17. Ministry of Health of Ontario, Women's Health Bureau.

Ornstein, M. (2000). *Ethnoracial inequality in the City of Toronto: An analysis of the 1996 census*. Access and Equity Unit, Strategic and Corporate Policy Division, City of Toronto.

Pajaczkowska, C., and Young, L. (1992). Racism, representation, psychoanalysis. In J. Donald and A. Rattansi, eds. *'Race,' culture and difference* (pp. 198–219). London: Sage.

Princeton Religion Research Center. (1987). *Religion in America*. Princeton, N.J.: The Gallup Poll.

Paris, P. J. (1995). *The spirituality of African peoples: The search for a common moral discourse*. Minneapolis, MN: Fortress.

Schreiber, R., Noerager, P., and Wilson, C. (1998). The contexts for managing depression and its stigma among Black West Indian Canadian women. *Journal of Advanced Nursing* 27, 510–17.

Sharma, N. (1994). July-Sept. Restructuring society, restructuring lives: The global restructuring of capital and women's paid employment in Canada. *Socialist Studies Bulletin 37*.

Stolley, J. M., and Koenig H. (1997). November. Religion, spirituality, and health among elderly African Americans and Hispanics. *Journal of Psychosocial Nursing and Mental Health Services 35* (11), 32–38.

Taylor, R. J., and Chatters, L. M. (1988). Church members as a source of informal social support. *Review of Religious Research 30* (2), 193–203.

Waldron, I. R. G. (2002). African Canadian Women Storming the Barricades!: Challenging Psychiatric Imperialism through Indigenous Conceptualizations of 'Mental Illness' and Self-healing. Unpublished doctoral dissertation, University of Toronto.

Wright, B. E. (1974). The psychopathic racial personality. *Black Books Bulletin 2*, 25–31.

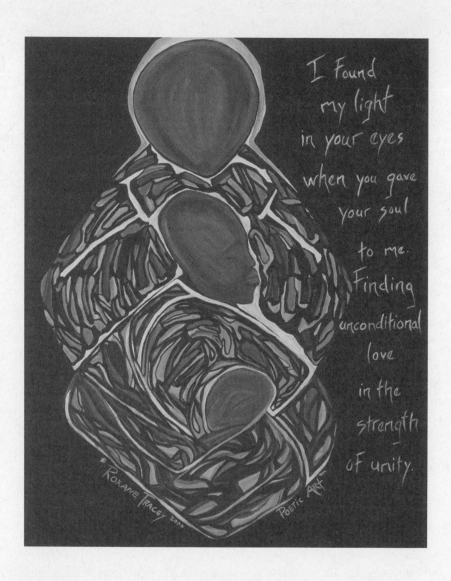

I Found my light in your eyes when you gave your soul to me. Finding unconditional love in the strength of unity.

© Roxane Tracey 2009

Poetic Art™

Think Globally, Act Appropriately: A Community Health Centre's Response to Violence Against Women in the Context of Black Women and Women of Colour

NOTISHA MASSAQUOI

It is Monday and, as usual, I begin my workweek leading a supervisory meeting with the mental health counsellors of Women's Health in Women's Hands. I enter our meeting room and notice in the far corner two suitcases neatly tucked out of the way. "Who's going on vacation?" I ask. We usually give weekend updates at the top of the morning, movies seen, parties attended, pet antics, anything to ground us before we go into the troubling details of our clients' lives. The suitcase, I was to learn, belonged to a client currently in an abusive relationship. The suitcases contained all of her valuable possessions and were being hidden in her counsellor's office for safe-keeping. When she was ready and able to leave her abusive partner, she would retrieve her belongings. As we began our session, it was hard not to notice those suitcases looming in the background. All of our work and the existence of our centre were metaphorically condensed into the images of two suitcases belonging to a victim of violence in the corner of a counsellor's office. What was contained in the baggage? Would she return? Even more important, what were the barriers preventing her from leaving an abusive life that would ironically compel her to place her valued material possessions in a safe space but not herself.

The physical context within which these thoughts occur is Women's Health in Women's Hands, a community health centre designed philosophically and architecturally to accommodate and address the health needs of Black women and women of colour, particularly those from Africa, the Caribbean, Latin America, and south Asia. Our multidisciplinary team of health care profession-als work from an inclusive feminist, anti-racist, pro-choice frame-work, and we believe that women have the right to receive quality health care and to make informed choices about their health. In fact, women are the experts in their health care and guide our process and our holistic services in order to address the barriers that prevent women from being healthy. The health care team in our idyllic centre consists of nineteen health promoters, nurses, doctors, health educator, dietitians, mental health counsellors representing fifteen countries and eleven languages, and in keeping with women glob-ally, one fifth of us have experienced abuse that was physical, sexual, and psychological in nature. More succinctly, I should say that one in five of the world's female population, including ourselves, has been physically or sexually abused by a man or men at some time in her life (WHO, 1994).

I include *us*, the health care professionals in these statistics, because we not only need to ground ourselves in the reality of the work that we do and the services we provide, but as a health centre that prioritizes Black women and women of colour, and is staffed predominantly by women from those same communities (a *for us, by us* strategy) we cannot afford to divorce ourselves from the women we serve. Not because we are now the workers does our experience of violence become irrelevant in the grand scheme of global violence against women. In fact, it is our ability to incorporate our personal experiences, professional knowledge, education, and our sometimes inability to divorce ourselves from the client who looks like us, sounds like us, and relates to us in ways that mainstream services cannot accommodate, thus creating a unique environment and perspective from which to address the issues, concerns, and strate-gies against violence gendered violence.

I may have been somewhat presumptuous to state that in light of the global statistics on violence against women one fifth of our staff have experienced some form of violence. It is in fact difficult to accurately measure the extent of gendered violence, and most would agree that a one in five statistic is a gross underestimation (WHO,

1999). For us at Women's Health in Women's Hands, violence against women is a commonplace issue that is addressed on a daily basis by all providers. When we look at our own statistics, for example, over the past year 70 per cent of the 146 clients who sought mental health counselling presented issues of violence and abuse in their sessions (Crawford and Massaquoi, 2000). The women we saw described experiences of dealing with abuse at the hands of strangers, the general community, but most commonly within their own families. They presented accounts of battering at the hands of husbands, partners, extended family members, sexual abuse of female children, trafficking and forced prostitution, sexual harassment at work and educational institutions, marital rape, female genital mutilation, and other practices harmful to women, forced abortions based on sex selection, battering during pregnancy, date rape, abuse of women with disabilities, and dowry related abuse.

The Declaration on the Elimination of Violence Against Women adopted by the United Nations General Assembly in 1993 defines violence against women as "Any Act of gender-based violence that results in, or is likely to result in physical, sexual, or psychological harm or suffering to women including threats of such acts, coercion or arbitrary deprivation of liberty whether occurring in public or private life (WHO)."

It is a definition that is able to encompass the broad range of experiences faced by our clients. But as one can see from the varied accounts of violence, understanding the prevalence, the expression, and the impact of violence on the lives of women becomes a difficult task.

The gross under-reporting of gender-based violence, particularly in the family setting, is a phenomenon in virtually every country globally. Statistics and reports available from the police, academic institutions, and women's organizations not only underestimate accurate levels of violence in women's lives due to under-reporting, but fail to capture or recognize violence based within a cultural context. We argue that culture will determine how women experience violence, how they name it, how they seek assistance – if at all, and how they are treated when they seek such services. Because definitions of violence are subjective and the Western women's movement often works from a narrow Euro-centric perspective, Black women and women of colour are often erased from the violence discourse. For example, common violence against women awareness raising campaigns highlight that a woman who is being physically, sexually, or emotionally abused needs help, and the fact that help is available is the prominent theme. How different would the target audience look if these campaigns also highlighted assistance for women being threatened with deportation, forced to work for unacceptable wages, forced into prostitution in the selection of options? Narrow definitions of violence which do not use a lens of race, class, and other forms of oppression, eliminate women of colour from the discussion, the statistics, protection, as well as the possibility of benefiting from intervention strategies to end violence against women.

I was hesitant to write this piece on behalf of WHIWH which looks at violence against women within the context of race, because it runs the risk of becoming the "race piece" as opposed to an organization's view of violence against women within the context of their philosophical framework. It also runs the risk of becoming a vehicle to perpetuate further the notion that violence against women is most prevalent in immigrant communities, families of colour are more violent, and our treatment of women within cultural contexts are oppressive and barbaric in comparison to the dominant White culture. In the mainstream context, violence in the lives of Black families and communities has become a normative practice, in part largely due to the biased media representations of the members of the community – particularly Black males (Collins, 1990). In domestic violence awareness campaigns, for example, the common rhetoric states that domestic violence can occur in a household despite race, educational level, and socio-economic status. As service providers, we all have an anecdote about the professional woman, with the wealthy husband, in an affluent neighbourhood, who was abused. We pull it out of our "you wouldn't believe it" bag in order to emphasize the prevalence of domestic violence in families, even upper middle-class White homes. The need to demystify the prevalence of violence against women in such households, and in essence ensure the protection of the women in these homes, has become the cornerstone of anti-abuse campaigns. To further this argument one would only have to promote such a disclaimer if the underlying assumption is that violence against women occurs predominantly amongst the poor, the undereducated, and within families of colour. This brings me back to my original point that focusing on violence against women without using an analysis of race or a racial lens maintains our gaze on, and the protection of, members of the White middle-class family at the expense of our own. To address the issue of violence against women in this manner ignores and endangers the lives of Black women and women of colour by failing to recognize their unique experiences of violence.

The Expanded Definition

Over the past two decades the modern women's movement has lobbied and organized against the commonplace violence that permeates the lives of women both publicly and privately. The backlash against violence that society exercises and condones against women represents one of the most salient and active forces for women's groups globally, their goal being to expose and prevent gender violence, most recently through the efforts to broaden the concept of human rights to include the right to be free from gender-based violence.

Gender-based violence, or the threat of it, is a social problem which takes many forms depending on the cultural context of the victim; from domestic abuse to dowry death, from sexual harassment in the work place to forced prostitution, from rape to involuntary sterilization. While all individuals are vulnerable to violence, this risk and, accordingly, the experience of violence is gendered and culturally expressed. In a conversation with a staff member at WHIWH, she noted that although she had no scientific evidence she had noticed that the number of domestic violence cases would increase during professional sporting playoff seasons. This is just as cultural as the increase of sexual assaults on women during military and political wars.

As a community health centre that prioritizes Black women and women of colour, we have had to adopt an expanded world view, and a resulting expanded definition of violence. It has been projected that the immigrant population in the city of Toronto where we are located will exceed 50 per cent of the total population by the year 2001 (Statistics Canada, 1995). It then becomes imperative for not only our centre to address issues that impact women from this perspective, but also organizations that have traditionally been accustomed to serving a mainstream clientele. The burden of servicing Black women and women of colour cannot only fall on ethnocultural agencies; allocation of resources makes this an impossibility. In order to ensure accessible, culturally appropriate services for all the women we serve, we have identified several areas that are crucial to consider in the address of violence against women.

Despite the fact that the past twenty years has been marked by resolutions, declarations, and conventions in support of women, and the year 2000 marked five years since Beijing, the adoption of a Platform for action which devotes an entire section to the issue of violence against women, violence against women remains a global issue. It is therefore not possible to address the issue of violence against women without addressing, and in our case challenging, the very nature of the socio, economic, cultural, political, and gendered ordering of society. It is not possible to address the issue of violence against women without acknowledging the truth that violence against women is supported and upheld in a system of racism, discrimination, and subordination. Without an expanded definition and response to gendered violence which takes into account the intersectional identities of Black women and women of colour, one which acknowledges the complexity of women's lives, validates women's experiences, understands the cultural, linguistic, racial, and class barriers embedded within in the structures of society and promotes an analysis which recognizes that violence against women is embedded in racist, sexist, homophobic, economic, and political discrimination, no women will be free from violence. This expanded worldview considers that it is necessary to situate gendered violence within a human rights discourse. The 1993 Declaration on the elimination of violence against women asserts that women are entitled to all human rights and fundamental freedoms, security and freedom from torture, cruel and inhuman and degrading treatment or punishment.

We have had to broaden our concepts of violence against women to reflect the complexities of women's lives, not only looking at violence that occurs within the confines of the family, but to also address violence within the community as well as offences by the state. Our work with immigrant and refugee women challenges us to increase our understanding of the increased risk of violence against women during armed conflict and displacement. For example, we need to look at rape not only as an act of power and control on a personal level, but also as a weapon of war and a weapon of genocide on a political level. We have had to look at the issue of the trafficking of women and sexual slavery (UN High Commission for Refugees, 1995) as well as the resurgence of FGM and other harmful practices against women in order for communities to reinforce cultural identity then under attack (WHIWH, 1998).

We have had to come to understand the need to view violence as a determinant of health, a factor or condition that is known to influence one's health. We understand that violence is a health issue and has far reaching consequences for women physically, emotionally, sexually, and reproductively. Strategies to improve the health status of women must address violence as a broad determinant of health as well as look at violence throughout a woman's entire life cycle, from sex selection at birth to elder abuse.

We understand that violence is most greatly exacerbated by poverty with Black women and women of colour often being the most marginalized. It is further compounded in environments of economic inequality between men and women where women lack decision-making power, and where there are restrictions on a woman's ability to leave the family setting due to racial, cultural, or linguistic barriers within society at large.

This expanded world view broadens the scope of the feminist political agenda, recognizing that confronting and incorporating all forms of violence into the struggle for human rights for all women is an imperative. Violence is the threat that links all forms of discrimination and subordination of women globally. Violence defined in this expanded form then promotes strategies that must address alternatives to poverty, increased access to educational opportunities, improvements in health care for women, and the barriers that prevent women from taking control over their lives.

Sexist Racism vs. Racist Sexism

Understanding the links between racism and gendered violence is a crucial component to any intervention strategy of note. In addition to the fear and financial constraints that dominate most battered women's lives, racial and cultural issues often even make it more difficult for Black women and women of colour to leave abusive relationships. In the context of violence against women, it must be noted that the violence that women experience is often shaped by the other multiple dimensions of their identities as women such as race class, ability, and sexuality. Feminist discourses often fail to acknowledge in particular the issue of race in the discussion of violence. In the same vein, discussions of gendered violence are often missing from discussions of racism as violence and its unique impact on women. Intersectionality then needs to be the framework within which we place the issues of gendered violence particularly as it impacts Back women and women of colour.

The concept of Intersectionality denotes the various ways in which race and gender interact to shape the multiple dimensions of Black women's lives (Crenshaw, 1991). The experiences of Black women and women of colour are frequently the product of intersecting patterns of racism and sexism constructed around negotiating interactions of subordination and oppression. Not to be represented accurately within the discourses of feminism and racism makes one think that all women are White and all Blacks are men. Because of their multiple identities as both female and of colour within discourses that demand prioritizing above an intersectional existence, women of colour are marginalized in both the world of the feminist and the anti-racist.

Why the Suitcases Remain: A Tale of Oppression

In the racially polarized world that Black women and women of colour exist, the challenge of maintaining the integrity of our families and communities often overrides the imperative of self-preservation. Many of us originate from cultures in which collectivism outweighs individuality, and the moratorium on exposing the private sphere is deemed crucial for the survival of the group. Unfortunately, this strategy of maintaining group cohesion places the onus on women to remain silent witnesses to the violence they experience in their lives, rather than on men to refrain from violent actions. The negative portrayals of Black people, in particular by the media, adds another factor which promotes the silence around issues of gender violence. We as Black people are constantly in the gaze of White society, and judged and stereotyped by the worst actions of our community members. The question then becomes how does the importance of our communities to be viewed favourably by the dominant culture become more valuable than living a life free from violence.

Audrey Smith and Sophie Cook are two names that encapsulate many of our worst fears about the violence experienced by Black women. For Black women it is not a far-reaching belief that the systems in place to protect women from violence fails in cases where Black women are concerned. In a frequently hostile, racist society, fear of protective services or law enforcement becomes a major deterrent in reporting acts of violence against women, and even a violent home becomes a safe haven from the racially hostile environment. Many of us women of colour come from communities where it is unheard of for the state to become involved in what is considered domestic affairs. Public intervention for many Black women involve the removal of Black children from Black homes, and in cases of women coming from military states or war torn countries this can be a fatal prospect. The securing of private, safe spaces at the expense of women's lives often becomes intensified by the racist environment that Black women and women of colour exist.

Support services such as sexual assault hotlines, women's shelters, and various women's organizations have been developed to ensure that victims of violence have safe, secure places to seek assistance. The assumption is often: (step 1) woman is abused, and (step 2) woman leaves home to seek safe shelter. For many women of colour, entering a women's shelter is the most disempowering event of their entire abuse experience, as opposed to the empowering framework that the shelter movement purports. The strategies of marginalization and subordination are often reproduced by the workers who, although they are women, hold positions of power over the clients in terms of information, resources, and freedom.

> When a White woman stood up for herself or demanded assistance in the shelter she was considered strong and well on her way to healing from the abuse. When a Black women does the same thing she is considered confrontational and hostile – *WHIWH client*

Women are often expected to abandon cultural practices in order to conform to the rules of the shelter. Barriers such as language, immigration status, lack of opportunities for education, and employment are not considered. The fact that women are often cut off from the cultural community during their stay in the shelter, compounded by marginalization and subordination often experienced within the shelter, can be as devastating as the violence these women escape. The fact that women of colour often do not fit culturally within the framework of the typical client from the mainstream, the myriad of services she would receive becomes the issue for the workers rather than ensuring that the services for all victims of violence are responsibly accessible.

In the case of immigrant women who have been sponsored, refugee women awaiting status, or women without status, the fear of the immigration process and deportation is ever present. An immigration system that remains inaccessible due to language barriers, a system which is not transparent and clearly biased against communities of colour, one that does not look favourably upon women with dependent children, or one that is financially inaccessible and often places difficult demands on women – such as proving self-sufficiency – places immigrant and refugee women, particularly those of colour, at risk for being abused by partners, abused by employers, and exploited at times by both (Crawford and Massaquoi, 2000). Even if a woman can prove sponsorship, breaking down the process of applying for the ministerial permit for humanitarian and compassionate grounds is a daunting experience at the least (McDonald, 1999).

My focus on the Intersectionality of race and gender in the discussion of violence against women by no means negates other oppressions experienced that are critical in shaping the experiences of women of colour. The point being made is that a discussion which does not at some point use race as a lens through which to analyze women's experience with violence will not ensure affirmative public positions and proposed strategies for elimination that can benefit all women.

Conclusion

The threat and reality of violence has become intertwined in the everyday life of women and, therefore, the everyday work of our staff at WHIWH. Violence is the consistent thread in all women's lives globally. Gendered violence limits a woman's ability to participate fully in society and care for herself and her family. It limits our choices as women, it compromises our health, it shortens our life span, erodes our self esteem, limits our mobility, and crushes our dreams. As we challenge ourselves as service providers we challenge our contemporaries to consider the following:

1. Recognize that violence against women is, first and foremost, a question of inequality and, by extension, a denial of human rights.
2. A more holistic approach to the understanding of violence is needed in order to design more effective prevention strategies and programs.
3. In order to prevent violence against women, society at large must mobilize to redefine many cultural, social, economic, and political processes.
4. Models of best practice within the health care system should be developed and shared.
5. Health care providers should address the exploration of personal biases and willingness to address violence in personal and professional life.
6. Screening of violence should be conducted with all clients.
7. Advocate for social infrastructure to provide women with the choice of seeking secure refuge and ongoing counselling that is culturally and linguistically appropriate.
8. Ensure that the intervention we bring into the lives of women suffering from violence does not undermine their sense of power, autonomy, and control over their own lives.

References

Brassileiro, A., ed. (1997). *Women against violence, breaking the silence, reflecting on experience in Latin America and the Caribbean*. United Nations Development Fund for Women (UNIFEM), New York.

Collins, P. (1990). *Black feminist thought*. New York: Routledge.

Crawford, C., and Massaquoi, N., (2000). When Mama sends for me; Immigration and the disruption of mothering. Paper presentation at the International Conference on Mothering in the African Diaspora. The Centre for research on Mothering, York University, Toronto.

Crenshaw, K. (1991). Mapping the Margins: Intersectionality, Identity Politics and Violence against Women of Colour. *Stanford Law Review 43*, 1241–99.

Health Canada and Kinnon Consulting. (2000), Women's Health – freedom from violence: practical tools.

Massaquoi, N. (2000). Writing resistance. In G. Sophie Harding (Ed.), *Our words, our revolutions: Di/verse voices of Black women, First Nations women, and women of colour in Canada*. Toronto: Inanna Publications and Education Inc.

McDonald, S. (1999). Not in the numbers: Domestic violence and Immigrant Women. *Canadian Women's Studies 3*(19) (pp. 163–167).

Statistics Canada (1995) Census Data.

White, E. (1990). *The Black women's health book: speaking for ourselves*. Seal Press, U.S.A.

Women's Health in Women's Hands. (1998). Policy position on female genital mutilation.

World Health Organization. (1994). Women's health: Towards a better future. Reporting of the first meeting of the Global Commission on Women's Health. Geneva.

World Health Organization (1999). Summary of international and regional human rights texts relevant to the prevention a redress of violence against women. Geneva, WHO.

World Health Organization (1997). Violence Against Women, Resource Booklet. Geneva WHO.

United Nations High Commission for Refugees. (1995). Sexual violence against refugees, guidelines on prevention and response. Geneva.

Black Women's Health in Nova Scotia: One Woman's Story

DR. WANDA THOMAS BERNARD

Introduction

This chapter examines Black women's health in Nova Scotia, beginning with a discussion of health and health process, then looking at health through the lens of oppression and interlocking oppressions. A brief commentary on systemic racism in the heath care system is provided, followed by an examination of the everyday reality of the interlocking nature of oppression. A brief history of Black women's activism work in Nova Scotia provides context for the conclusion of the chapter, a discussion of the impact of racism and oppression on Black women's health, and the implications for Black women's health care.

In this chapter, I present a case study using a clinical narrative to examine the impact of race, gender, and class oppression on the health and well-being of an African-Nova-Scotian woman. Her story is told through the life cycle stages and critical incidents that were defining moments for her. Narrative inquiry provides a way to understand experience (Clandinin and Connelly, 2000, p. 20). Involving collaboration between researcher and participants, narrative inquiry is both the living and telling of stories. Using narrative inquiry in this case provided me with an opportunity to hear this woman's story to better understand her experience. This enabled me to give her perspective on the meaning, relevance, and importance of these life events. Cortazzi (2001) asserts that telling stories of personal experiences is a way of looking at and evaluating the past. My evaluation of this case enabled me to develop much better understanding of our health care system and Black women's experiences of accessing health care.

Health and Health Process

Any discussion of health needs to begin with a working definition of health. I use the World Health Organization's (WHO) definition, which states that "health is a state of complete physical, social, and mental well-being, and not merely the absence of disease and infirmity." (Baxter, 1990, p. 3.) Clearly, a holistic definition of health is very complex, and this becomes most visible when undertaking health research. This examination of health introduces the concept of health as a process and, more specifically, looks at the impact of the interlocking nature of oppression from the standpoint of Black women.

Cowley and Billings (1999) discuss three ways to view health: health as a product, health as potential, and health as a process (p. 995). They go on to suggest that health is a continuing pattern of change occurring over a lifetime in all dimensions of the individual (Anderson in Cowley and Billings, p. 995). Viewing health as a process fuelled by the accumulation and use of resources for health, Cowley and Billings (1999) conclude that the process of building capacity is more important than the presence or absence of specific resources. Furthermore, they posit that a sense of coherence, or a pervasive, enduring and dynamic feeling of confidence that things will work out, is firmly rooted in the context of the individual. As defined below, this sense of coherence has three dimensions: comprehensibility, manageability, and meaningfulness (Cowley and Billings, 1999, p. 996):

Comprehensibility: the perception of a stressful situation as structured and explicable;
Manageability: the confidence in one's ability to meet the demands of the stressful situation, which depends on their faith and access to various resources, or a sense of self-empowerment;

Meaningfulness: the belief that stressful situations are worthy of
investigation and are purposeful challenges (Antonsvsky in
Brooks, 1998, p. 234).

According to Cowley and Billings (1999), individuals do have the
ability to make sense of their experiences and to understand those
events at an emotional and cognitive level; however, their argument
does not take into account the impact of structural realities on individuals' lives and on the process of health.

Health Canada (2001) identifies the following key determinants
of health:

- Income and social status
- Social support networks
- Education, employment/working conditions
- Social environments
- Physical environments
- Personal health practices and coping skills
- Healthy child development
- Biology and genetic endowment
- Health services
- Gender and culture

One's social location in relation to the matrix of these determinants of health will dictate, to a certain extent, the health process of
individuals, regardless of individual will and determination. More
recently, researchers have linked issues of sexism and racism to the
health and well-being of Black women (Association of Black Cardiologists, 1999; Enang, 2002; Women's Health in Women's Hands,
2000). Enang (2002) argues that policies based on the determinants
of health and the social inclusion framework may help address
complex Black health issues, such as the impact of racism on health
and health process (p. 52). A critical appraisal of the health process,
the determinants of health, and one's ability to make sense of one's
own reality is rooted in an understanding of the impact of multiple

and interlocking oppression on individuals. Brooks (1998) argues that a sense of coherence is central to one's ability to successfully cope with events that pose a threat to one's health. However, this does not take into account the fact that one's sense of coherence can be seriously compromised by one's experience of racism and oppression. I have stated elsewhere that one of the greatest travesties of racism for people of African descent is that it causes victims to give up, with no sense of hope or entitlement (Bernard, 1996). This is further influenced by the impact of interlocking oppression, as our social identity and social location helps to shape and define our experiences and responses to those experiences. To experience that "sense of coherence" that Cowley and Billings (1999) refer to, an African-Nova-Scotian woman would need to be able to critically analyze her health status and health process from the location of oppression, and gain some agency in that process.

Reflections of Health from the Location of Oppression

The term *oppression* emphasizes the pervasiveness of inequality in social institutions, and of that which is entrenched in our individual consciousness. According to Thompson (1993), oppression often involves disregarding the rights of an individual or group. Thus, one's *location* will bring differential treatment, or the process of *othering*, which makes possible the denial of equitable access to the goods and services offered by organizations and institutions. Looking more specifically at the social construction of health, Abrums (2000) highlights how one's social location affects one's definition of health and healthy behaviour. Similarly, Beardslee's (1989) study is a good illustration of the impact of race and class oppression on health. For women of African descent, gender oppression becomes an additional burden (Bernard, Lucas-White and Moore, 1993; Enang, 2001; Gordon, 2002). Other research that has examined the relationship between health and socio-economic status (Baxter, 1990; Fick and Thomas, 1995; Hay, 1994; Sharif, Dar and Amartunga, 2002) emphasizes the impact of economic disadvantage on both health status and access to health care. There has also been much research examining the impact of gender on health (Coleman, 2000; hooks, 1993; van Roosmalen, Loppie and Davidson, 2002; Taylor, 1999); however, little research has been conducted on African-Canadian women's health (Enang, 2002). Such research would need to examine the interlocking systems of oppression rooted in racism, sexism, classism, ageism, heterosexism, and ableism, and their short- and long-term impact on health and well-being. These issues are explored in this chapter through the narrative of one African-Nova-Scotian woman's experience of the health process and access to heath care.

To be marginalized from the mainstream based on race, poverty, gender, a combination of these, or other interlocking oppressions, is to feel exclusion on a daily basis. Class is often the glue that helps to keep oppressive structures intact (Bishop, 1994). People marginalized by poverty know that this exclusion goes beyond economics, and includes systemic exclusion from life's everyday amenities that many take for granted. Black women are disproportionately represented amongst the economically disadvantaged in Nova Scotia (Hamilton, 2000). In addition, Black women are more likely to experience triple jeopardy (Bernard, Lucas-White and Moore, 1994) as they grapple with the conditions that affect them, based on their race, gender, and socio-economic status. The most visible of these conditions is the impact of systemic racism on health care for African-descended people. To fully understand and address exclusion, we need an informed analysis of the systemic policies and practices that help to maintain the oppression and deprivation of the economically oppressed. Furthermore, an analysis of their impact on health is essential if we are to improve health care services for these marginalized groups.

SYSTEMIC RACISM IN HEALTH CARE
There has been little documentation on the topic of racism in the health care system in Canada; however, we can learn from the experiences of our colleagues in America. For example, a compelling article entitled "Racist Health Care: Reforming an Unjust Health Care System to Meet the Needs of African-Americans," Vernellia R. Randall (n.d.) asserts that:

Wounded, racism retreated to more subtle expressions from its most deeply entrenched bunker.... Forms of sophisticated racism attached to economic opportunities unfortunately can still be found today.... [However,] nowhere is that better exemplified than in the rate of excess death among African-Americans.

Throughout our painful history in the West, African people have endured the tremendous burden of oppression imposed by pervasive institutionalized racist practices. We also know that our survival has come at the expense of our health and our quality of life. From the beginning of our existence on the American continent, people of African descent have been subjected to unfair medical treatment. The story in Nova Scotia is no different. African-Nova-Scotians are not represented at the policy and senior management levels of the health care system, but are certainly over-represented in those who are facing serious and life-threatening health issues. Because of the cumulative effect systemic racism has on the lives of African-Nova-Scotian people, they are likely to face (Ali, n.d.):

- High risk of depression and suicide
- Feelings of helplessness, hopelessness, fear, mistrust, despair, alienation, and loss of control
- Damaged self-esteem
- High risk of addictions and violence
- High stress and more stress-related illnesses such as high blood pressure, heart disease, and problems of the nervous system
- Poor general health and depressed immune systems
- Short lifespan
- High infant death rates
- High unemployment, underemployment, low wages, and unsafe working conditions
- Limited access to jobs, housing, education, and the services they need to be healthy.

Today, Africans throughout the diaspora feel the pandemic sting of HIV and AIDS. Conditions such as sickle-cell anemia, or G6PD (Glucose-6-phosphate dehydrogenase deficiency), diseases particular to African-descended populations, prostate cancer, diabetes, fibroids, and many more diseases continue to have inadequate funding for research, screening, testing and, in almost all cases, a cure. Recent research conducted on the health care needs and issues affecting the African-Nova-Scotian community (Bernard, forthcoming; Black Women's Health Group, 1998; Enang, 1999) also substantiates the existence of systemic racism. Enang (1999) asserts that the lack of culturally appropriate services, and the lack of screening for diseases that are common to African people, are examples of the ways in which the health care system systematically discriminates against members of the African-Nova-Scotian community. Similar claims come from the Black Women's Health Group, which asserts that access to health care services is negatively affected by systemic barriers in employment and transportation. For example, the material reality of the interlocking nature of systemic racism means that a poor unemployed Black woman in Yarmouth County may have more difficulty getting early detection and treatment for breast cancer than a woman in a similar situation in Halifax. This interlocking nature of oppression is explored in the case study of Tanya.

A BRIEF HISTORY OF BLACK WOMEN IN NOVA SCOTIA

A brief historical account of Black women's experiences in Nova Scotia will help set the context for the case study. The first presence of African people in Nova Scotia dates back to 1605 (Pachai, 1990). However, it was not until the early 1800s that a significant African presence in Nova Scotia was made possible through "a number of segments traceable to slaves, Black Loyalists, Maroons, and Black Refugees" (Pachai, 1990, p. 61). While each cohort came from different and distinct locations in the African diaspora, each helped to create what we now know as African-Nova-Scotian society. One significant thing that each group shared was relegation of people of African descent to the bottom of the social and economic hierarchy (Christensen, 1998; Pachai, 1990). These people also learned to live and cope with the shame and stigma attached to the legacy of slavery and, as Christensen (1998) argues, "Blacks who obtained their freedom were only marginally better off than slaves. The history of oppression has been costly to Black Canadians" (p. 43). The emotional and psychological well-being of African people has been severely influenced by this history of oppression and marginalization from the mainstream, or what Christensen (1998) calls the "cycle of unequal access" (p. 54). The resultant impact on Black women's health is further explored in the case study.

While much of the history of Black people in Nova Scotia renders Black women invisible, it is important to note their work, especially their activism, that helped to create pathways to empowerment for the community as a whole. From a historical perspective, Black women's involvement in racial uplift in Nova Scotia can be found in the work of women like Dr. Pearleen Oliver and Dr. Carrie Best. Oliver may be best known for her work in the African United Baptist Association (AUBA) with her husband, the late Dr. William P. Oliver; however, her greatest influence may be her work to challenge systemic racism in the nursing profession. Through Oliver's intervention, racial barriers in nursing schools were challenged, allowing Black students to study nursing (Hamilton, 2000). This led to racial uplift in two specific ways. First, it meant that young Black women could consider nursing as a career, thereby, challenging traditional roles that would see them destined for work in-service; that is, in the residential and/or commercial cleaning industry. Secondly, it meant that a Black nurse could treat those who would use health care services for the first time in Nova Scotia's history. The impact of Oliver's initiative is still experienced today.

Dr. Best's activist work took place in a different arena. In 1947, Best began the *Clarion*, Nova Scotia's first Black newspaper. In addition to her work in publishing the *Clarion*, Best also wrote for the *Halifax Herald*, the *Pictou Advocate* and the *Nova Scotia Gleaner*, making the needs and concerns of Black Nova Scotians visible to a much wider audience. Through this medium, Best was able to promote a more balanced reporting of issues seen as significant and important by the Black community. As Sadlier (1994) asserts, as an investigative reporter, Best was widely recognized as a strong advocate for and the voice of the Black community in Nova Scotia. Best worked untiringly to help "uplift the race," and this work has been recognized locally and nationally.[1] Best's own autobiography, *The Lonesome Road* (1977), is a telling story of Black women's activism, highlighting the struggles, barriers, acts of resistance, and empowerment that form part of the legacy she has left for the next generation of social activists.

As Bernard, Lucas-White, and Moore (1993) posit, the Black communities of Nova Scotia have produced many strong women who have contributed much to the survival of the group (racial uplift) (p. 272). Profiling some of those contributions and empowerment strategies helps to bring others along and facilitates the self-determination (Bernard, 1996) of sister warriors in the struggle. Self-determination is the ability to define ourselves, name ourselves, create for ourselves, and speak for ourselves, and here refers to women's self-empowerment and actions that facilitate such practices. Black women's involvement in their families, churches, and communities may best illustrate their activism in this area. Black women have also been described by others as the strength of their communities and families (Bernard, 1996). Many authors and writers have documented the role of Black women as "superwomen" (Bernard, Lucas-White, and Moore, 1993; Collins, 1990; Hamilton, 1982; hooks, 1981; McCray, 1980). There is also evidence in the literature of Black women's activism in Nova Scotia that is rooted in the theme of self-determination (Black Cultural Centre for Nova Scotia, 1987, 1990; Hamilton 1982, 1994). One could begin with the work of Rose Fortune, from Annapolis Royal, who was the first woman police officer and business owner in Nova Scotia. An escaped slave, Fortune is the epitome of self-determination. She began her own transport business in 1825, and business ownership was a tradition that her family carried on for generations.[2] Fortune's early involvements in male-dominated work are remarkable examples of feminism and self-determination in action. The legacy of her work lives on in the work of her extended family and community.

Similarly, evidence of social change can be found in the early work of the AUBA, and the women's work within that organization. While the AUBA was formed in 1855, women did not go as delegates until 1891, and the women's work was not officially organized until 1895 (Hamilton, 2000). The formation of the provincial women's group, named the Ladies Auxiliary, did not happen until 1917, and the Women's Institute did not begin formal meetings until 1956. Clearly, although women were involved in the AUBA since its inception, their work would not be recognized until much later in this male-dominated organization. The male-dominated leadership and inherent sexism in the AUBA has been recognized by others as well (Bernard, Lucas-White, and Moore, 1993; Hamilton, 2000). Despite this legacy of unnamed sexism and patriarchy, the AUBA has enjoyed tremendous support from all sectors of African-Nova-Scotian society. The AUBA has always been primarily a spiritual organization; however, it has also had a mandate to deal with the social, educational, economic, and political issues of the Black community. Staying with this tradition, when the women's group was organized, its mandate included the following four key issues: sick, charity, membership, and social reform (Hamilton, 2000). Hamilton (2000) notes that the social reform committee was instructed to "observe well racial conditions, and bring them before the auxiliary in order that the executive of the association may deal with such questions" (p. 40).

As previously noted, the determinants of health have a significant impact on one's health and one's ability to make sense of the health process when one is faced with a health crisis. Caught in a spiral of oppression, struggle, and resistance, Black women have a number of obstacles to overcome in order to maximize their sense of health and well-being, and to have access to adequate health care. From a history of slavery and oppression has developed a legacy of strength and survival among Black women. Although issues of systemic racism in health care have had a devastating impact on Black women's health in Nova Scotia, Nova Scotian women have survived. The case study discussed in the remainder of this chapter is an example of how one can achieve victory over struggle.

I use the case study of Tanya[3] to explore some of the challenges that a Black woman living with race, gender, and class oppression faces when trying to access the health care system, and to get culturally appropriate services. I trace Tanya's experience from birth to death, expanding on critical health incidents that framed her entire existence.

BEGINNINGS

Tanya's life course was scripted at birth in the late 1950s in Nova Scotia. She was a Black child born to a single-parent mother, Brenda, who was mentally challenged and blind. Tanya was her fifth child, and although her extended family had cared for the others, they felt they could not care for another baby. The child welfare authorities determined that Brenda could not possibly care for this child on her own; therefore, they placed the baby in permanent care and custody of the department of child welfare.

A Black child born in the 1950s had significant challenges to overcome because of the historic and endemic racism that affected the education, housing, employment, and life circumstances of Africans in Nova Scotia. To be a child in need of care and protection placed an additional challenge on Tanya, and her life course was shaped by circumstances beyond her control. We see here the beginning of the interlocking nature of oppression rooted in racism, sexism, classism, and ableism, and the effect of this oppression on this individual.

Initially, Tanya was placed in a White foster home in Halifax, as the agency did not have any approved Black foster homes.[4] However, within two years the foster mother died quite suddenly, and in the absence of finding another home on short notice, Tanya was placed at the Nova Scotia Home for Coloured Children, where she remained until age four. Tanya was moved to another White foster home at that time, as the social worker believed Tanya would do better in a smaller family environment. At that time, Tanya was described as withdrawn and prone to fits of anger. She appeared to be developmentally delayed, as her speech lagged behind others in her age group. A psychological assessment indicated that she had not adjusted to her environment. Tanya's own words aptly describe the challenge that she faced as a child and the way in which the system began to fail her:

Tanya said, "I never knew my mother, or why I was taken from her. I never believed that my own mother could ever treat me as bad as my foster mother did, so why did they take me from her?"

A race analysis of this case might have led the agency workers involved to make different decisions regarding Tanya's care. For example, McRoy (1991) suggests that agencies carefully assess foster families prior to placement to determine if they would be a suitable permanent placement. This would decrease the number of placements children have, and allow them to develop a secure attachment without having to transfer attachments to a new caregiver. McRoy (1991) includes the ability to foster a positive racial identity among the factors that should be examined in a foster home assessment. She argues that attempts should be made to place Black children with Black families or with extended family members. However, when this is not possible, placement agencies must consider the social and racial environment in which the child will be socialized. In addition, McRoy (1991) suggests that all foster families should receive training on post placement services and the development of positive racial self feelings in Black children, a view that is shared by the Association of Black Social Workers (ABSW Position Statement, 1989).

THE MIDDLE CHILDHOOD YEARS

At the tender age of four, Tanya was moved to her third placement, the Moshers. The professionals who were responsible for her wondered why she had delayed development and difficulty adjusting. What was planned as a positive move to a family setting actually became a nightmare for Tanya. While this new home had two parents, a stay-at-home mother, other Black foster children Tanya's age, and all the amenities, it was not a safe and nurturing environment for her. From the first day she arrived at the Mosher home, Tanya experienced emotional and physical abuse by her foster mother

– who also abused the other children in her care – and sexual abuse by her foster father. Her foster mother called Tanya racist names, told her she was unworthy, and beat her whenever something went wrong; she also blamed Tanya for the misbehaviour of all of the children. Tanya was expected to model positive behaviour for her foster siblings, so when they acted up, she was punished along with them. Tanya's foster father simultaneously showered her with affection and attention in public, while sexually abusing her in private, telling her she was "special" so she got "special treatment." Tanya was confused by the sexual abuse and responded with mixed feelings, because her foster father was the only person who seemed to give her any positive attention in comparison with the horror of the emotional and physical abuse by her mother. It is easy to understand how she would see this form of abuse as positive and affirming. He was the one person who made her feel special. This was later to become the most difficult aspect of Tanya's history for her to deal with.

The signs that Tanya was an abused child were clearly present, but the social workers and teachers that she came into contact with missed them. She was failing in school, had many unexcused absences, was aggressive, withdrawn, and had low self-esteem. By the time she was twelve, she was also visiting the doctor frequently because of recurring urinary tract infections. Although these signs were present, they were all treated as isolated incidents; therefore, the abuse went unnamed and there was no intervention to help Tanya. The health care system did not question or investigate why this young girl had so many infections. The child welfare system also missed an opportunity to intervene in Tanya's life at this critical point. While Tanya had multiple exposures to health risks, these were identified as her own individual problems and not externally controlled. This persistent exposure to violence would later have a significant impact on Tanya's beliefs and attitudes toward her own health, when she said: "After a while I believed that I deserved to be abused and that all check kids got treated that way.... The abuse was so bad and everybody knew about it, but nobody did anything about it.... I thought it was normal." Fick and Thomas (1995) assert that there is a relationship between exposure to violence and the shaping of healthy beliefs and behaviour in economically disadvantaged children.

THE TEEN YEARS

The teen years were probably the most challenging for Tanya. Between the ages of thirteen and seventeen, she had four medically approved abortions, and was labelled promiscuous during this period. Each time she became pregnant, her foster father took her to the doctor and arranged for the abortion. No one questioned the number of pregnancies. No one inquired about the fathers. The health care system and the social welfare system failed Tanya, because no one treated her holistically. No one expressed concern about the multiple pregnancies or the school absences. She was labelled sexually promiscuous, but no one looked for the cause of this behaviour. While it is hypothesized that adolescents with histories of abuse are more likely to engage in adolescent risk-taking behaviour, and that poverty is associated with a higher prevalence of chronic health conditions (Davidson and Manion, 1996), these issues were not seriously investigated in Tanya's case.

Meanwhile, Tanya continued to be sexually abused by her foster father, and the physical abuse by her foster mother was becoming more serious. When Tanya was hospitalized for a broken arm, the foster parents said she fell down the stairs. On another occasion, she sought medical treatment for a dislocated shoulder. By this time, there was growing awareness in the community that the foster children in the Mosher home were being abused; however, this was never reported to the authorities, as it was assumed that no one else would take these poor Black children. The Moshers were affirmed in their community for their willingness to care for these children who might otherwise be in an institution. So the abuse continued, and Tanya became increasingly depressed. She had had no contact with her birth family, and by the time she was eighteen, the Moshers were the only family she knew. In Tanya's mind, her foster siblings were her real siblings, and so were her foster parents. She had developed a love/hate relationship with her foster parents, which was to become a major hurdle for her in later years. As Tanya frequently told me, the love that she felt for her "family" was the one thing that helped her get through the crises in her life, yet it was also that love that enabled the abuse to continue.

Tanya recalled that "the only person who ever loved me was Dad [foster father] so I learned to tolerate the abuse so that he would not stop loving me.… I also had to protect my younger [foster] sisters from him."

GRADUATING FROM FOSTER CARE

To reach the age of eighteen in foster care is a significant milestone. Termed "graduating from care" by many of the youth themselves; this is the time when cases are terminated, unless the child is continuing in higher education. By the time Tanya was eighteen, she had already dropped out of high school, as she could not cope with the name-calling and ridicule to which she was subjected. On her eighteenth birthday, Tanya's social worker visited, for what was to be the last time, to inform her that she was now of age and free to go on her own. This was devastating news for Tanya, as she had nowhere to go. She had a grade ten education and had had no preparation for independent living. She was also five months pregnant, and had not told anyone because she did not want to have another abortion.

Tanya was frightened and, after her social worker left the home, swallowed a bottle of her foster mother's medication in a desperate plea for help. This was considered a serious suicide attempt; therefore, Tanya was certified mentally ill and admitted to the local psychiatric hospital. Not unlike her previous access to health care, the mental health system also failed Tanya. Although they treated her depression, they failed to address the underlying problems that led to the suicide attempt. In addition, they made referrals to local services for young single mothers to help her deal with the pregnancy, but no effort was made to provide services to the father, or to even find out who he was. This led to my first contact with Tanya.

As a social worker in the mental health setting, this case was referred to me for follow up. As a Black woman, I certainly recognized some of the issues around race, class, and gender she was struggling with that had contributed to her current situation. However, I failed to understand the issues of violence and abuse that had framed her reality for the past fourteen years, and their impact on her mental health. My immediate goals were to reconnect Tanya with the Black community and her birth family, and to help her in independent living, but she needed much more from the health care system. Tanya needed to deal with the issues of physical, emotional, and sexual abuse that she had endured for years from the people who were paid to care for her. In addition, she was being thrust into the role of mother, when she still needed to be mothered herself. She was being supported to live on her own, to connect with the family that had abandoned her in the first place, and to leave the comfort of the only family she knew, even though they had been so abusive. This was all under the auspices of *helping* in the health care system. The system was not meeting all of Tanya's needs, partly because the system did not identify those needs. When the health care system fails to treat people from a holistic perspective, then it will fail to meet those people's needs. Tanya was thrust into adult roles and responsibilities when her development had arrested at a pre-adolescent stage.

ADULTHOOD AND THE RESPONSIBILITIES OF PARENTING
Within a few months of graduating from care, Tanya was not only adjusting to independent living and being totally responsible for herself for the first time in her life, but she was also now responsible for her infant daughter. Child welfare authorities re-entered her life as they tried to provide supports to her as a young single mother. I continued to see her in outpatient mental health, but the focus was very much on managing daily depression, and the underlying issues were not addressed as they were not seen as priorities. These unresolved issues, however, led Tanya to make some poor decisions and choices that had a very negative impact on her life. Furthermore, one could ask how Tanya could be expected to get on with her life without dealing with those issues that had interrupted her development. Caught at the intersection of race and gender oppression,

Tanya was also trapped in a cycle of poverty, low self-esteem, and self-abusive behaviour. There was no hierarchy of the oppressions that she embodied. Because these issues were not dealt with, Tanya went from one crisis to another, constantly running from the *real* issues.

Tanya got involved with a young man soon after her daughter, Susie, was born. The relationship seemed to go well at first, but once Tim moved in with them, Tanya was again subjected to severe physical and emotional abuse. Each time Tanya was abused, she relived the years of abuse she suffered in her foster home. She plunged further into depression and, as a result, found it difficult to care for her child. She also began using drugs as a way to cope with her pain. The cycle of abuse, depression, drug abuse, and suicidal ideations was to continue until Susie was four years old, and Tanya was readmitted to the psychiatric hospital. Susie was taken into care and placed with Tanya's foster parents, who had offered to help. There was no other community or family support, since her connection with her birth family had not worked out. Tanya's unresolved anger and blame created insurmountable barriers for her, and when distressed, she retreated to the *safety* of the family she knew.

This was my second point of contact with Tanya. We had a major breakthrough during this admission to hospital. Tanya disclosed her history of abuse for the first time and, to her surprise, she was believed. Her daughter, Susie, was immediately removed from the Mosher foster family, and placed with a member of Tanya's extended family. Tanya went into long-term therapy to deal with the past issues of abuse and trauma in her life, and the current issues of depression and drug abuse. I have noted elsewhere (Bernard, 2002) that women who struggle with drug addiction are often dealing with a number of issues, and Black women in Nova Scotia, especially, have few resources to help them, and this was certainly the case with Tanya. She made excellent progress, however, and was eventually able to regain custody of her daughter. This was a new beginning for Tanya, as she was now prepared for the responsibilities of adulthood and motherhood. For the first time, Tanya said she was "able to face the real demons in my life.... I finally learned that I did not have to take the abuse anymore when I realized that I put my little girl at risk. I want things to be different for her."

A NEW BEGINNING AND THE END

Tanya was beginning to feel very good about herself and was managing her responsibilities quite well. She was enrolled in an academic upgrading program to improve her employability skills. She was actively involved with Susie's school as a volunteer, and they were both engaged in community activities. For the first time in her life, Tanya felt a sense of self-esteem, self-determination, and empowerment, and could imagine a good future for herself and her child. No one was prepared for the physical health crisis that would be Tanya's next challenge, but her new-found sense of agency, empowerment, and purpose helped to guide her decision-making.

Tanya had discovered a lump in her right breast. She kept this terrible news a secret for months because she feared the authorities would take her daughter again; however, as the pain became unbearable, she eventually told me about the lump. I accompanied her to the doctor and she was immediately referred to a specialist. Further tests revealed that the lump on her breast was malignant, and that it was a secondary cancer. The main tumour was on her lungs, and inoperable. This was devastating news. Tanya was given six months to live, when she had really just begun to have a life.

Tanya was hospitalized shortly after the diagnosis; however, her condition quickly deteriorated. She was a poor, single mother of an eight-year-old child. She lived in public housing and had little flexible income and a limited support system; however, she approached this health crisis with a different perspective. She had an analysis of the issues that framed her life and she was determined to make decisions that would create a different pathway for her daughter. She had survived many other health crises in her life, and was finally able to claim self-recovery (hooks, 1993) from trauma. Finally, I could see a sense of coherence (Cowley and Billings, 1999) in Tanya. Tanya had two wishes: to die at home, and to ensure that family cared for her daughter. One of the last things she said to me was: "Wanda, I don't want my daughter to become a check kid.... I cannot allow that to happen to her."

To ensure that Tanya received the best possible culturally relevant holistic care during this end-stage of her life, I organized a case conference. She needed pain management and twenty-four hour care. Health care budgets could not cover all the costs. A group of church, extended family, and community volunteers were recruited and trained to provide for Tanya's care at home, supported by the palliative care team. Plans were put in place to find a permanent home for Susie within their extended family. At this end-stage of life, Tanya was able to comprehend her life story and make sense of the issues that had haunted her for years and, to her surprise, the health and social systems were finally working together to provide the best care for her. We did the right things for her in the end, and Tanya did die at home and in peace, knowing that her daughter, Susie, would be cared for by a cousin who had agreed to adopt her.

Conclusion

Tanya experienced multiple oppressions throughout her life, which interlocked on many levels. She was simultaneously marginalized and/or oppressed by her race, gender, and class, her location as a foster child in care, and her health status as a person with mental health difficulties. Her health was adversely affected by most of the determinants defined by Health Canada (2001). Part of Tanya's everyday reality was her struggle to survive this web of oppression and her relative marginalization from mainstream society. Her health was a continuing pattern of change occurring in all dimensions over a lifetime (Cowley and Billings, 1999). Furthermore, both the health care and the child welfare systems failed Tanya from her birth. Assumptions were made about her birth mother's ability to provide for her care because she was developmentally delayed and blind. Was this decision rooted in discriminatory attitudes about persons with disabilities and their ability to parent? Why was there no contact with Tanya's birth family? Were there efforts to reconnect her to her birth family at age two, when her first foster mother died? Perhaps things had changed in the family. Why was this not an option for Tanya?

The abuse that Tanya suffered in her last foster home could have been detected at a number of points, by the health care system, the school, the community, or the child welfare system. There were many clues that were missed or ignored. As well, access to adequate health care was clearly limited for this young Black person who was being raised by White parents. What assumptions were made when her White father took her for the repeated abortions? Black women are sexualized at an early age. Poor women are also stigmatized. Do such assumptions cloud professionals' judgement when assessments are conducted? What was the impact of racism, poverty, and gender on Tanya's ability to get adequate health care?

This case has haunted me for most of my professional career, and it has been somewhat cathartic to discuss it in this forum. I have frequently asked the questions that are presented here. The one area that I have learned from most is the interlocking nature of oppression and how intervention strategies need to account for this. During my first contact with Tanya, I was not aware of the significance of intersecting oppressions, and operated with an analysis that assumed that race and gender were the two most salient issues to be addressed. This focus affected the type of assessment I was able to do. It was not holistic; hence, important issues were missed. Race and gender were important and certainly contributed to the conditions that she lived with, but these were not the only issues that needed attention. I was fortunate to have had another opportunity to intervene in Tanya's life and provide a more relevant service to her. At the most critical time in her life journey, we were able to help her meet her health and social needs, because we knew what those needs were. By taking control of the situation and by becoming her case manager, I was able to direct her health care plan. As Tanya coped with her last struggle, she was finally empowered (Evans, 1992; Pinderhughes, 1983) to demand the service that she wanted for herself. This was made possible because the health care professions were finally able to share their power with her.

Reflecting back on this case, I would suggest that, to successfully navigate the health care system, one needs an advocate, preferably one who is situated within the system, or who is very knowledgeable about it. Culturally relevant holistic care for Black women should be the norm, not the exception. Efforts are currently under way in Nova Scotia to ensure that Black women get better health care services, and lessons learned from this case can help in that process. The Black Women's Health Group, the Health Association of African-Canadians, Cancer Care Nova Scotia, this writer and others are currently engaged in research and community outreach projects aimed at improving health care access and services for Black women and their families. They are identifying barriers and strategies for change to improve systems like those that Tanya came into contact with. Such changes would honour the struggles that Tanya and other women like her have endured and survived.

Endnotes

1   Best has an honorary doctorate of law degree from St. Francis Xavier University and has been appointed as both a member and officer of the Order of Canada (Sadlier, 1994).
2   Daureen Lewis is a great-niece of Rose Fortune. Lewis is former mayor of Annapolis Royal, owner of a local business, and currently heads up the Women and Business Centre at Mount Saint Vincent University, helping other women develop their business careers. She is one of the women featured in *Black mother black daughter*.
3   The names in this case study have been changed to protect the identity of the individuals involved. The issues in the case are taken from an actual case that I worked with; however, some of the situations have been adjusted to protect anonymity.
4   The experience of race and racism in the adoption and fostering of a Black child is examined in Folaron and McCartt-Hess (1993); Hutchinson and Pepin (1994); Mallows (1989); and Twine (1999).

References

Abrums, M. (2000). "Jesus will fix it after awhile: Meaning and health." *Social Science and Medicine 50*(1), 89–105.

Ali, S. n.d. "Racism and health." Retrieved [November 1999] from http://home. ican.net/~edtoth/ndphealthrac.html.

Association of Black Social Workers. (1989). Position Statement. Unpublished document. Halifax, N.S.

Baxter, M. (1990). *Health and life styles*. New York: Routledge.

Association of Black Cardiologists (1999) Black Church Women Develop Strategies to Reduce Risk of Heart Disease, Presentation made to the National Association of Social Workers Annual Conference, April 1999, Atlanta Georgia.

Beardslee, W. R. (1989). The role of self-understanding in resilient individuals: The development of a perspective. *American Orthopsychiatric Association 59*(2), 266–76.

Bernard, W. T., Lucas-White, L., and Moore, D. (1993). Triple jeopardy: Assessing life experiences of Black Nova Scotian women from a social work perspective. *Canadian Social Work Review 10*(2), 256–76.

Bernard, W. T. (1996). Survival and Success: As Defined by Black Men in Sheffield, England and Halifax, Canada. Unpublished doctoral thesis. Sheffield: University of Sheffield.

— (2000). Beyond Inclusion: Diversity In Women's Health Research. Keynote Address. In *Proceedings of the MCEWH Atlantic Provinces Policy Forum* (pp. 153–82). Halifax, N.S.

— (2002). Including Black women in health and social policy development: Winning over addictions. In C. Amartunga (ed.), *Race, ethnicity and women's health* (pp.153–82). Halifax, N.S.: Atlantic Centre of Excellence in Women's Health.

Best, C. (1977). *That lonesome road: The autobiography of Carrie M. Best*. Nova Scotia: Clarion.

Bishop, A. (1994). *Becoming an ally*. Halifax: Fernwood.

Black Cultural Centre for Nova Scotia (1987). Traditional Lifetime Stories: A Collection of Black Memories. Vol. 1, Dartmouth, Black Cultural Centre for Nova Scotia.

Brooks, J. D. (1998). Salutogenisis: Successful ageing and the advancement of theory on family caregiving. In McCubbin , and Hamilton, I., eds. *Stress, coping and health in families: Sense of coherence and resiliency* (pp. 227–48). Thousand Oaks, CA: Sage.

Christensen, C. (1998). Social welfare and social work in Canada: Aspects of the Black experience. In V. R. D'Oyley and C. E. James, eds. *Re/visioning Canadian perspectives in the education of Africans in the late 20th century* (pp. 36–57). North York: Captus Press.

Clandinin, D. J., and Connelly, F. M. (2000). *Narrative Inquiry*. San Francisco: Jossey-Bass.

Coleman, R. (2000). Women's health in Atlantic Canada: A statistical portrait. In *A portrait of women's health*, Vol. 1 (pp. 9–42). Halifax, N.S.: The Maritime Centre of Excellence for Women's Health.

Collins, P. H. (1990). *Black feminist thought*. New York: Routledge.

Cortazzi, M. (2001). Narrative analysis in ethnography. In P. Atkinson, A. Coffey, S. Delamont , J. Lofland and L. Lofland, eds. *Handbook of ethnography* (pp. 384–93). London: Sage.

Cowley, S. and Billings, J. R. (1999). Resources revisited: Salutogenesis from a lay perspective. *Journal of Advanced Nursing 29*(4), 994–1004.

Davidson, S., and Manio, I. G. (1996). Facing the challenge: Mental health and illness in Canadian youth. *Psychology, Health and Medicine 1*(1) 41–56.

Enang, J. E. (2002). Black women's health: Health research relevant to Black Nova Scotians. In C. Amartunga, ed. *Race, ethnicity and women's health* (pp. 43–82). Halifax, N.S.: Atlantic Centre of Excellence in Women's Health.

— (1999). *The childbirth experiences of African Nova Scotian women*. Unpublished master's thesis. Halifax, N.S.: Dalhousie University.

Evans, E. N. (1992). Liberation theology, empowerment theory and social work practice with the oppressed. *International Social Work 35*, 135–47.

Fick, A. C. and Thomas, S. M. (1995). Growing up in a violent environment: Relationship to health-related beliefs and behaviours. *Youth and Society 27*(2), 136–47.

Folaron, G. and McCartt-Hess, P. (1993). Placement Considerations for Children of Mixed African-American and Caucasian Parentage. *Child Welfare 72* (2), 113–25.

Fraser, R. and Reddick, T. (1997). *Black women's health: Final report*. Halifax, N.S.: North End Community Health Centre.

Gordon, Debra. (2002), May 15. African American women and menopause. http://www.intelihealth.com.

Hamilton, S. (1982). Our mothers grand and great: Black women of Nova Scotia. *Canadian Woman Studies 4*(2), 32–37.

— (1994). Naming names, naming ourselves: A survey of early Black women in Nova Scotia. In Bristow P., Brand, D. Carty , L., Cooper, A., Hamilton, S., and Shadd, A., eds. *We're rooted here and they can't pull us up: Essays in African Canadian Women's history* (pp. 13–40). Toronto: University of Toronto Press.

— (2000). *African Baptist women as activists and advocates in adult education in Nova Scotia*. Unpublished MA Thesis, Halifax, N.S.: Dalhousie University.

Hay, D. I. (1994). Social status and health status: Does money buy health? In B. Singh Bolaria and Rosemary Bolaria, eds. *Racial minorities, medicine and health* (pp. 9–52). Halifax, N.S.: Fernwood.

Health Canada. (2001). What determines health? Retrieved (30 October 2001) from www.hc-sc.gc.ca/hppb/phdd/determinants/e_determinants.thml

hooks, bell. (1981). *Ain't I a woman: Black women and feminism*. Boston: South End Press.

— (1993). *Sisters of theyam: Black women and self-recovery*. Toronto: Between the Lines.

— (1994). *Teaching to transgress*. New York: Routledge.

Hutchinson, Y. and Pepin, M. (1994). Multicultural/Multiracial Policy as it relates to Placement of Black Children in Foster Homes. *The Social Worker 62*(4), 185–89.

Mallows, M. (1989). Abercrave weekend: exploring the needs of transracially adopted young people. *Adoption and Fostering 13*(3); 34–36.

McCray, C. A. (1980). The Black woman and family roles. In Rogers-Rose, ed. *The black woman* (pp. 67-78). Thousand Oaks, CA: Sage.

McRoy, R. (1991). Significance of ethnic and racial identity in inter-country adoption within the United States. *Adoption and Fostering 15*(4), 53–60.

Pachai, B. (1990). *Beneath the clouds of the promised land*, Vol. 2. Halifax, N.S.: Black Educators Association of Nova Scotia.

Pinderhuges, E.B. (1983). Empowerment for our clients and for ourselves. *Social Casework 64* (June), 331–46.

Randall, V. R. n.d. Racist health care: Reforming the health care system to meet the needs of African Americans. Retrieved (30 November 1999) from http://www.udayton.edu/~health/pages/racial.htm

Sadlier, R. (1994). *Leading the way: Black women in Canada*. Toronto: Umbrella Press.

Sharif, N. R., Dar, A. A., and Amaratunga, C. (2002). Ethnicity, income and access to health care. In C. Amartunga, ed. *Race, ethnicity and women's health* (pp. 121–52). Halifax, N.S.: Atlantic Centre of Excellence in Women's Health, Halifax, N.S.

Taylor, J. Y. (1999). Colonizing images and diagnostic labels: Oppressive mechanisms for African-American women's health. *Advances In Nursing Science 21*(3), 32–45.

Thompson, N. (1993), *Anti-discriminatory practice*. London: MacMillan.

Twine, F. W. (1999). Transracial Mothering and Antiracism: the case of White Birth mothers of Black children in Britain. *Feminist Studies 25*(3), 729–74.

van Roosmalen, E., Loppie, C., and Davidson, K. (2002). Women's voices: Atlantic Canadian women's contribution to health policy. In C. Amartunga, ed. *Race, ethnicity and women's health* (pp. 15–42). Halifax, N.S.: Atlantic Centre of Excellence in Women's Health, Halifax, N.S.

Women's Health in Women's Hands. (2000). Personal communication with program director from Women's Health in Women's Hands, Halifax, N.S.

Misogyny and Mental Illness

CARLA R. RIBEIRO

The disproportionate numbers of women among the ranks of mental patients, and the pathologization of socially encouraged patterns of female behaviour, speak volumes of the rampant misogyny of our culture. In this paper I will demonstrate how psychology as a discipline is implicated in the process by which such a notion becomes entrenched in popular consciousness. Women are no more "mad" than men, but misogyny works to convince us all that this is true. With its eurocentric, masculinist focus, the discipline of psychology is implicated for its role in the construction of a feminine identity that creates a double bind for most women. In a now famous study, Broverman et al. (1970) found that the profile of the mentally healthy adult fit much more closely with the profile of the mentally healthy male. What this suggests is that characteristics typically associated with women are, by definition, less healthy than those typically associated with men.

Major psychological theorists and practitioners are also accountable for their theories and therapies that have ignored the multifaceted cultural, structural, and interpersonal forces affecting individual functioning and development, and have formalized the concept of "blaming the victim." The key players in the American Psychiatric Association who hold the power to define who is normal and who is not, must also be held accountable. I will expose the very political and unscientific nature of the Diagnostic and Statistical Manual (DSM) decision-making process. As we shall see, the process of psychiatric diagnosis and categorization is deeply flawed and loaded with implicit assumptions about sex roles. Focusing on DSM disorders with which women are disproportionately afflicted, dependent personality disorder, self-defeating personality disorder, multiple personality disorder, eating disorders, depression, I argue that the symptoms of these are normal responses to the physical and psychological abuse that many women undergo on a daily basis at the hands of individual men, patriarchal institutions, and states. However, in order to understand the theoretical justification for gender bias in the diagnosis and treatment of women, we must first become familiar with the major theoretical schools of personality development.

Feminist Critique of Major Psychological Paradigms of Normal/ Pathological Personality Development

> [T]raditional, or mainstream, personality theories and views of psychopathology are not adequate from the standpoint of feminist theory. This inadequacy is found in a number of areas in the traditional theories – in their limited views of human nature; their exclusion of multiple internal and structural forces affecting human development and functioning; their narrowly constructed definitions of mental health and mental disorder, a result of dominant group collaboration; and ultimately, their underlying intellectual processes. (Brown and Ballou, 1992, p. xi)

The study of normal personality and pathology has been a major preoccupation of the discipline of psychology. Numerous theories have been put forward: some have fallen into disrepute and been discarded, and some persist and have earned their way into psychology textbooks. An examination of these traditional theories is important because they have played a paramount role in defining how we think about psychological phenomena, and have greatly influenced our taken-for-granted conceptions of mental health. Feminist psychology has provided both a new understanding of women and a critique of the old theories that neglected to include women's lives in their analyses. As we shall see from the theories that I will examine in this paper, classical theorists tended to focus on nature/nurture dichotomies, ignoring the role of variables such as gender and diversity in personality development.

Laura Brown and Mary Ballou (1992) propose a new standard by which to judge personality theories and their accompanying definitions of pathology. By adding gender and diversity to the list of variables to be evaluated, they have asserted that content cannot be divorced from context in understanding who we are, what we do, and why we do it. They propose an evaluation of personality and psychopathology based on analyses of complex, interlocking, often overlapping variables. In other words, it is an oversimplification to view mental disorder as exhibiting monocausality (i.e., originating in a single cause). It is more appropriate, given the layers of complexity of human social life, to view mental disorder as being, in Freudian terms, overdetermined or having more than one cause. The major thesis of Brown and Ballou's work, as stated in the epigraph at the beginning of this section, points to the tendency of mainstream psychology's focus on the individual to obscure the dominant ideology embedded in its theories. Brown and Ballou and the other contributors to their book, call for theories of personality and psychopathology that are set in the context of "the multifaceted cultural, structural, and interpersonal forces affecting individual functioning and development." (Brown and Ballou, p. xii). According to them a feminist analysis "requires multidisciplinary perspectives that articulate these forces, which describe the full range of human characteristics, kinship patterns, and political/social/economic/historical arrangements" (Brown and Ballou, p. xii). The following is a very brief overview of the major approaches to personality and psychopathology and some of the problems associated with each. What is presented here is by no means an exhaustive analysis of all theories of personality and psychopathology within each major approach. While there have been significant modifications and improvements within each paradigm, some of the underlying assumptions remain the same. These are under examination in this paper.

Of all psychological grand narratives, Freud's psychoanalysis has perhaps received the most criticism from feminists for being both misogynist and phallocentric. Freud's major theoretical propositions in relation to personality are that the unconscious mind is a major determinant of behaviour, and that sexuality is present from birth and plays a key role in the formation of individual identity. He theorized that the early experience of the child and the successful resolution of each stage of psychosexual development – oral, anal, phallic, and genital stages, especially the resolution of the Oedipus complex – lay the foundations for the adult personality. Unsuccessful resolution, coupled with the constant battle for dominance between aspects of the unconscious mind, resulted in neurotic anxiety, which he saw as the heart of psychological disturbance. Of all Freudian theories, the one which has perhaps received the most criticism is his Oedipus complex theory of personality development. Much has been written about this controversial theory, but here I focus my attention on how it relates to female personality development.

Psychoanalysis argues that women are biologically disadvantaged because of their lack of a penis, a deficiency they realize during the Oedipal stage of development and for which they subsequently blame their mothers. The prognosis for female personality formation is therefore dismal at best, since the resolution of the Oedipus complex and formation of the superego is a crucial prerequisite for healthy adult functioning.[1] The story goes something like this. When the young girl first becomes aware of her lack of a penis she begins to feel like she is missing something. As this feeling intensifies (penis envy) she begins to feel hostility towards the mother whom she presumes is responsible for her deficiency. She rejects the mother and turns to the father for love. Since the little girl can hardly give up the mother in real terms, she tries to replace the mother's essence within herself by identifying with her and by trying to take the mother's place in relation to the father. Freudians believe that girls do not reach as conclusive a resolution to the Oedipus complex as do boys, primarily because such resolution is motivated by the intense fear associated with castration complex. Since girls believe that castration has already occurred, it does not provide the same motivational force for them. The result is an inferior super-ego which makes women biologically, emotionally, morally, and spiritually inferior to men and therefore forever incapable of realizing their full potential. This phallocentric view of women's psychology, based entirely on inference, has done nothing to understand female personality development from the standpoint of women.

As a theory of personality, traditional psychoanalysis is lacking for several reasons. First, its model of universal personality development assumes and is based on the heterosexual nuclear family with the mother as primary caregiver. How are we to understand personality development in societies whose dominant family form is other than the nuclear family? Are we to assume that people raised in single parent or lesbian and gay households have not developed full personalities? Secondly, psychoanalytic theory has only really considered female development as an add-on to male development. Freud developed his theory of (male) personality development first and later adapted it to apply to women. Needless to say, such an approach can never provide a fair treatment of female psychology. Thirdly, the psychoanalytic notion of the powerful unconscious does not seem to include internalized societal messages about what it means to be Black or White, male or female. It does not consider how those forces work intrapsychically and, often, unconsciously, to limit human development.

There has been and still needs to be much feminist critique and revision of Freud. It is beyond my purpose to examine those here, since I want to focus specifically on the traditional Freudian perspective, as it is understood by a wider population of academics and lay people alike.

Behaviourism

Behaviourism in psychology has its roots in the work of Ivan Pavlov, John Watson, and B. F. Skinner. Behavioural theory on personality emerged out of implied and applied conclusions resulting from an understanding of learning principles; the major contribution of this school of psychology. Behaviourism posits that all behaviour is learned, determined by the environment, and shaped by its consequences. In this model, there is no free will, but merely individuals responding in specific ways to specific stimuli. What is learned, therefore, can be unlearned. Behaviour that is considered undesirable or maladaptive (a term advanced by Skinner) can be extinguished simply by manipulating the stimulus-response contingency. Internal aspects of behaviour are not considered and emotions are seen as involuntary behaviour. As is often the case when paradigms shift, behaviourism is a response to what was considered lacking in its predecessor, psychoanalysis. Its strong adherence to the principles of scientific positivism can be seen as a direct rebellion against the metaphysical, unscientific nature of psychoanalysis.

While behaviourism has had a powerful effect on academic psychology, it has serious limitations when applied to personality. Firstly, it trivializes, ignores, and/or dismisses such phenomena as compassion, trauma, cultural or gender beliefs, moral, cognitive, and affective development in the construction of personality. Secondly, it implicitly uses normative criteria to arrive at definitions of what is adaptive or maladaptive. This model is inadequate for several reasons. Fundamentally, it clearly fails to address the diversity and richness of human experience. Complex human processes are reduced to what can be measured or observed. Another key failure of behaviourism is its unwillingness to consider and challenge environmental stimuli. It accepts external stimuli as givens and places the onus to change on the individual. For example, it is not enough to expose women to assertiveness training without challenging the cultural beliefs and practices that, on the one hand, produce women as passive victims and, on the other, men as perpetrators of violence against women. There is nothing in behaviour therapies that suggest sensitivity to issues of gender, race, and class, which are important determinants in many women's lives. Nor does it make explicit its reliance on the cultural norms and values of the dominant group in its assessment of adaptive, healthy behaviour. Furthermore, its reliance on a simplistic cause-effect model privileges rationality as the only ordering principle of human behaviour. Here I refer not to philosophical notions of rationality as a cognitive process, but to the rationality implicit in the notion that all human beings will always seek to maximize pleasure and minimize pain. This does not begin to appreciate the complex, intrapsychic war that is waged between gender expectations, personal desires, and cultural norms for a woman's behavioural response.

While social cognitive and cognitive-behavioural theorists (e.g., Albert Bandura, John Dollard, Albert Ellis, George Kelly) have begun to pay closer attention to the complexities of the individual and the role of internal processes, the key issues mentioned above are still, by and large, being ignored.

Humanistic/Phenomenology

The humanist personality theorists (e.g., Carl Rogers, Frederick Fritz Perls, and Abraham Maslow) in psychology emphasized the wholeness of human experience and postulated that human choice, intentionality, and awareness fundamentally influence our actions. In general, they focused on personal experience and the individual's perceptions of those experiences as the major determinants of behaviour. Humanists developed their theories primarily out of their clinical work with clients. It is no surprise, then, that humanistic psychology is also associated with psychotherapy that is often described as *non-directive* or *client-centred*. Although there are differences among humanist theorists, I will explore some of the central arguments of this viewpoint and discuss how they are inadequate concerning women and other oppressed groups.

Rogers has suggested that reality is what is perceived by the individual, as opposed to some external, objective reality that exists in spite of the individual. This is perhaps the greatest limit of the phenomenological approach to human experience. While I agree that, in some instances, reality is what is perceived through the senses, as a woman of colour I know too that reality is not wholly determined internally. The external reality of racism and sexism for me present real obstacles, regardless of my perception of them. If I have a strong internal locus of control, then I may make certain choices regarding how to get around those obstacles. No doubt these choices can and will affect my reality, but the reality is that racism and sexism have already limited the kinds of choices I can make.

Maslow's theory depicts a hierarchy of needs. He begins with physical needs and ends up with emotional and spiritual needs. Maslow's postulate is that once the needs of one level of the hierarchy are met then the individual can move into the needs of the next level up, and so on, until self-actualization occurs. While Maslow's needs pyramid is potentially useful, I wonder if he has considered how it is that large portions of the human population will never get beyond the lowest levels of physical needs. Does this mean that these people are inferior "persons" or does it mean that they live in environments that deny the satisfaction of their basic needs? Maslow provides no answer to these questions.

From a feminist standpoint, humanistic personality theories are attractive because they have focused on personal experience. This emphasis is absent from the other two major theoretical approaches – Freudianism and behaviourism – and thus was initially welcomed in feminist and psychological circles. But they do not go far enough. They have failed to recognize how influential external forces really are. Most of us who are feminists now know that patriarchal institutions limit and severely constrict the possibilities for women, regardless of whether those women perceive their situations as oppressive or not, whether they themselves feel empowered or not. Any examination of the lives of women as a whole does not allow us to conclude that, once we have made it through Maslow's hierarchy and find ourselves actualized, we will live free from physical and psychological abuse from our environment. Contrary to what is implied in humanistic theory, a woman cannot simply change her perception of herself and consequently, magically eliminate all the cultural, legal, economic, and social obstacles to her actualization.

The preceding discussion of the major theories of personality is by no means exhaustive and is at times, admittedly, oversimplified. It is beyond the scope of this paper and, therefore, not my intention here to provide an exhaustive analysis and critique of psychology's treatment of women. What I have tried to do is focus on the three major traditional schools of psychology, and show why they have been lacking with respect to female psychology. Although some of these theories have been modified, such a discussion remains valid because the major issues remain. In the next section, I will discuss the process by which psychodiagnostic typologies are created and applied. I will also discuss some of categories of disorders that are typically associated with women, and show how these can be seen as normal, adaptive behaviour to what are essentially oppressive conditions.

Diagnosis, DSM and Women's Disorders

No more, I will accept no more
    be sorry no more
be quiet no more
They will have to hear my story
and they will not dare to say it
    made me mad
Of course it made me mad
After all they pathologised
    my history
No more, no more
my shouts today will be
    so loud
My tears drop of pure fire
you will no longer take away
    my past
for today I take my life
into these hands

I am a time-bomb
and I have started ticking (Walkerdine, 1990, p. 160)

Currently, the most influential tool used by psychiatrists, psychologists, and other mental health practitioners is the American Psychiatric Association's (APA) Diagnostic and Statistical Manual of Mental Disorders. This is a very important book, which can be regarded as the bible of the mental health industry. It plays a key role in mental health practitioners', as well as lay people's judgments about who is normal and who is not. I know first-hand the scope of the DSM's influence, since I first learned about the DSM diagnoses as an undergraduate student in an Abnormal Psychology class. I also know, as Caplan (1987) has pointed out, that the courts, hospitals, and insurance companies generally recognize its diagnoses. It is crucial then to understand how the creators of the DSM arrive at their decisions regarding who is normal and who is not. In the last decade or so, a great deal has been written about the methods and techniques used in this process. Before looking at some of that literature, it is first useful to review a brief history of the DSM process.

The first DSM was published in 1952 and only listed a few dozen types and subtypes of mental illness (Larkin and Caplan, 1992). By 1980, with the publication of DSM-III, the number had increased dramatically to over two hundred types and subtypes. The DSM-III and DSM-III-R (1987) were spearheaded by Dr. Robert Spitzer, a psychiatrist at Columbia University who selected nineteen psychiatrists, psychologists, and epidemiologists who, in turn, were responsible for recommending members of twenty subcommittees organized for the purpose of studying various types of mental disorders. This number seems small, especially when one considers the significance of the task of defining normalcy and pathology. Caplan has also pointed out that the APA has historically been made up of male psychiatrists. Currently less than 15 per cent of its membership is female (Larkin and Caplan, 1992). It is not surprising then that the DSM has been a site of institutionalized misogyny, since the vast majority of its authors and consultants have been White male psychiatrists who have tended to define themselves as "normal" and those who differ from them as "abnormal."

Caplan (1991) has provided significant insight into the way in which the process of revising and updating the DSM works. She and others (Rosewater, 1987; Walker, 1987) have exposed the generally unscientific, sexist nature of the DSM decision-making process in their specific discussions about the Self-Defeating Personality

Disorder (SDPD) controversy. It is important to review some of that debate here.

SDPD, originally named *masochistic personality disorder*, first appeared in DSM-III-R (1987) in spite of much public protest. Much of the criticism centres on the fact that SDPD pathologizes the average, traditional woman and the victim of abuse. Many of the diagnostic criteria for SDPD ("... rejects opportunities for pleasure or is reluctant to acknowledge enjoying him- or herself ... fails to accomplish tasks crucial to his or her personal objectives ... engages in excessive self-sacrifice that is unsolicited by the intended recipients of the sacrifice ...") fit the image of normal women, who conform to the traditional, socialized feminine role. Other criteria of SDPD ("... chooses people that lead to disappointment, failure, mistreatment even when better options are available ... rejects or renders ineffective the attempts of others to help ... following positive personal events ... responds with depression, guilt or behaviour that produces pain ... is uninterested in or rejects people who consistently treat him or her well ...") characterize the coping strategies of survivors of abuse (learned helplessness) (Caplan and Gans, 1991). In response to these concerns, the DSM authors added two clauses to the diagnosis, explaining that it could not be applied to women who were either depressed or in abusive situations. However, as feminist therapists like Rosewater (1987) have noted, most therapists do not inquire about their clients' history of abuse, and clients do not offer the information. Although SDPD was included in the Appendix as a category requiring further study, this decision was made even in light of evidence that suggested that there was not an adequate empirical base for the diagnosis, as well as evidence of serious methodological problems with the data that *had been* collected. Lenore Walker (1991) sums up:

> During the SDPD debates in 1985/86 the psychiatrists, primarily male, listened politely to the presentation of the research that demonstrated the bias against women, and confusion with normal stereotypical behaviour

encouraged in women that was presented by the criteria for SDPD.... Then they thanked the mostly female researchers very nicely, and went on with the creation of the categories anyhow (p. 137).

Caplan (1987) criticized the APA for failing to meet its own standards when it included SDPD in DSM-III-R. According to DSM-III (APA, 1980) categories could only be included if they were soundly based in good research, minimized subjectivity in the decision to apply a particular category to a particular patient, and were atheoretical. The research base on which the SDPD decision was made was very small, including only two studies of very small and dubious samples. The first study was limited to psychodynamic therapists in a single hospital setting (Rosewater, 1987). The second consisted of a questionnaire mailed to a select group of psychiatrists (APA members who had an interest in personality disorders) who were asked whether or not they believed that SDPD should be included in DSM-III-R. If they answered yes, they were instructed to complete the rest of the questionnaire. If they responded no, they were not required to complete the rest of the questionnaire (Caplan, 1987). Caplan (1987) points to the biased sample and the fact that even though half of the APA members polled did not believe that SDPD should be included in the DSM-III-R, it was included anyway. Rosewater (1987) also noted that the SDPD criteria excluded only current victims of abuse, even though long-term victims present the same characteristics. She further suggested that some SDPD criteria also ignored the patriarchal context in which many women live. For example, in the context of a society where women are encouraged to put their families first and engage in work that is unpaid, underpaid, and devalued, and where women earn less than men even when they do the same work as men, women in abusive situations must weigh the options of staying and putting up with the abuse or leaving and living in poverty. From this perspective, staying or leaving may be seen a lose-lose proposition.

The profound sexism inherent in the practices of the APA and the DSM process has also been demonstrated in the response of the

DSM-IV Revision Task Force to the category *delusional dominating personality disorder* (DDPD), which was proposed by Caplan and Eichler in 1989 (Larkin and Caplan, 1992). The proposed category is characterized by:

> inability to establish and maintain meaningful inter-personal relationships and identify and express a range of feelings in oneself ... inability to respond appropriately and empathetically to the feelings and needs of close associates and intimates ... tendency to use power, silence, withdrawal, and/or avoidance rather than negotiation in the face of interpersonal conflict ... having excessive need to inflate the importance and achievements of oneself, males in general, or both ... a tendency to feel inordinately threatened by women who fail to disguise their intelligence ... an inability to derive pleasure from doing things for others ... tends to characterize leaders of traditional mental health professions, military personnel, executives in large corporations, and powerful political leaders of many nations but can be found in all social strata and religious and ethnic groups. (Caplan and Eichler, cited in Pantony and Caplan, 1991, p. 121).

This category, which was developed primarily for the purposes of education and consciousness-raising, was also submitted to the APA Task Force in the hope that the lack of balance in the DSM could be addressed, and also to encourage the APA to recognize the harm and danger that results from rigid or extreme forms of traditional masculine behaviour (Pantony and Caplan, 1991). These authors pointed out that the DSM's inclusion of a category that pathologized the extreme, traditional feminine role alongside the absence of any parallel category for its masculine counterpart, exposes the tendency of the mostly male institution to define behaviour with which they identify as normal and those with which they do not, as pathology. Larkin and Caplan (1992) have identified what they refer to as "DSM gatekeeping techniques" used to exclude serious consideration of the DDPD category. It is useful to restate those here since they shed light on the ways in which sexism is translated into practical obstacles that harm women and limit their potential contributions. These gatekeeping techniques, which are derived from correspondence between Caplan and the Task Force members, include:

> questioning the seriousness of Caplan and Eichler's intentions in proposing DDPD as a diagnostic category ... saying they would review the empirical work (on DDPD) if Caplan and Eichler would assemble it, although their own people do the literature reviews for other categories ... refusing to specify the exact standards and criteria which they use in deciding whether to include or exclude categories ... dismissing with no explanation Caplan's point that there is a great deal of existing research which is relevant to DDPD ... explicitly discouraging the DDPD authors by following up on a comment about the need for Caplan and Eichler to provide empirical support for DDPD with a statement that, "if this sounds discouraging, I'm afraid it is meant to ..." Insinuating that the DDPD authors would not *want* to provide them with the empirical support for DDPD, although they had offered to do so ... dismissing DDPD before seeing the relevant review of the literature ... failing to assign a Task Force member to coordinate the review of the DDPD category ... stating that they were against adding new diagnostic categories ... claiming to be unaware of research relevant to DDPD, although the DDPD authors had informed members of the DSM-IV Revisions Task Force about that research and mentioned bodies of literature in a letter to them ... dismissing the research on violence against women, attribution theory, and many other topics as irrelevant to DDPD while continuing to include research on "masochism" as "support" for SDPD despite the differences in criteria for masochism and SDPD. (p. 22)

The inclusion of SDPD in DSM-III-R and the exclusion of DDPD from DSM-IV unmask the inherent sexist bias that underscores the DSM process. DDPD has not been pathologized because it characterizes the behaviour of the powerful men in our society who possess the ultimate power to define normalcy. It also exposes the political nature of the process that directs DSM decisions and calls into question the "scientific basis" of those decisions. I have spent a great deal of time discussing the DSM process of deciding who is normal and who is not. Using this discussion as a stepping stone, I will now examine some of the other disorders with which women are disproportionately afflicted – personality disorders such as multiple personality disorder (now called dissociative identity disorder), dependent personality disorder (DPD) and self-defeating personality disorder (SDPD), depression and eating disorders such as anorexia and bulimia – and further demonstrate how the process of psychiatric diagnosis and categorization is deeply flawed and loaded with implicit assumptions about sex roles.

Personality Disorders

Dependent personality disorder (DPD) is marked by "a pervasive pattern of dependent and submissive behaviour beginning in early childhood and present in a variety of contexts" (Spitzer and Williams, 1987, p. 347). As is the case with SDPD, this description fits closely with what we are *supposed* to be as women. This is consistent with the findings of Broverman and others that suggests that if women succeed in their role as women they may be diagnosed as having a personality disorder. Kaplan (1983) exposes the inherent sexism in this diagnosis by pointing out that dependency in men – relying on others to maintain their houses and take care of their children – does not receive a diagnosis as a disorder. Similarly, self-defeating personality disorder (SDPD) is defined as "a pervasive pattern of self-defeating behaviour, beginning by early adulthood and present in a variety of contexts. The person may often avoid or undermine pleasurable experiences, be drawn to situations or relationships in which he or she will suffer, and prevent others from helping him or her" (Spitzer and Williams, 1987, p. 371). One could argue that the vast majority of women who engage in heterosexual relationships with men are suffering from this disorder!

Multiple personality disorder, now renamed dissociative identity disorder (DID) is perhaps the most serious of those I discuss here. It is described as "[t]he existence within the person of two or more distinct personality or personality states.... At least two of these personalities or personality states recurrently take control of the person's behaviour" (Spitzer and Williams, 1987, p. 272). This is clearly a problem because of the confusion and psychological distress involved in having multiple personalities compete for control of one's body. However, it is crucial that we ask the following questions? What are the situations that give rise to such a disorder? Is this behaviour abnormal in those situations? There is very strong evidence to suggest that DID is causally related to child abuse. Putnam and others (1986) found that of a hundred people suffering from DID, 83 per cent reported sexual abuse. Repeated physical abuse was reported in 75 per cent of the cases, and the witnessing of violent death during childhood, usually of a parent or sibling, was reported by 45 per cent of participants. An extremely high incidence of child abuse in women diagnosed with DID strongly suggests that it is to be understood as a way of coping with or denying the trauma associated with such abuse. Here I would suggest that DID is a *normal* response to an extremely pathogenic life situation. This does not mean that sufferers do not need help, care, and counselling to deal with their fragmented lives. However, this approach would pathologize the situation rather than the individual and would rightly place scrutiny at the source of the problem – a misogynist culture.

Depression

According to Russell (1995), depression is the most common psychiatric diagnosis and has been received by women in disproportionate numbers. It is an emotional state in which a person feels unhappy.

The symptoms may be many and varied and include: "loss of interest or pleasure in almost all usual activities, poor appetite or weight loss or increased appetite or weight gain, insomnia or hypersomnia or other sleep disturbances, psychomotor agitation or retardation, decrease in sexual drive, loss of energy, fatigue, feelings of worthlessness, self-reproach or excessive and inappropriate guilt, difficulty in thinking and concentrating, persistent restlessness and irritability and suicidal thinking and/or attempts" (Spitzer and Williams, 1987, pp. 218–22, 229). While there is no doubt that women in large numbers are chronically unhappy, I question the usefulness of labelling them as mad or ill. I agree with Wiener and Marcus (1994) who have argued that the concept of depression individualizes a social problem: "[h]elplessness, powerlessness, and worthlessness do not occur in social vacua" (p. 225). As with personality disorders, the diagnosis functions to encourage women to situate their problems in relation to their own pathology, rather than a society that is in need of change. Phyllis Chesler (1972) in her classic work, suggests:

> women *do* get "depressed" as they grow older – when their already limited opportunities for sexual, emotional, and intellectual growth decrease even further.... Women are in a continual state of mourning – for what they never had – or had too briefly, and for what they can't have in the present, be it Prince Charming or direct worldly power (pp. 43–44).

As the search for a biological basis for depression continues, it is somewhat *depressing* that women's unhappiness can only be taken seriously if we can understand it in scientific terms.

Eating Disorders

If we rely on the DSM definition of eating disorders, most women who live in North American society suffer from eating disorders, albeit to varying degrees. "Intense fear of gaining weight or becoming fat" and "[p]ersistent overconcern with body shape and weight" plague most of us (Spitzer and Williams, pp. 67–69). While a search for a genetic/endocrine component to eating disorders is underway, I do not accept that eating disorders represent an extreme shift from the patterns of most North American women's lives. What is the context of women's lives that makes it necessary for them to engage in what Eva Székely (1988) calls the "relentless pursuit of thinness." In a society where women are psychologically assaulted daily by media images that dictate what we should look like, feel like, be like; where underweight blond, blue-eyed models are presented as the epitome of female beauty, it is a small wonder that so many of us will go to any length necessary to look like these models. This is compounded by the fact that many of us have internalized the notion that a woman's most significant asset is the way she looks. All of us, regardless of what we do, are viewed by society as women first, inhabiting our imperfect women's bodies. Székely points to the pressures women face to be thin in order to gain a job, keep a job, get a man – the right kind of man, and so on. The message is that we will be rewarded for our efforts to lose weight and stay thin by success in both our professional and personal lives. It is interesting to note that eating disorders do not exist or are extremely rare in some socio-cultural contexts that are unlike our own. It has also been found that they only exist in the context of plenty (Lee et al., 1989). What all of the above points to is that eating disorders are a direct by-product of a body-conscious culture, obsessed with thinness. Women are the main casualties, and it is not surprising that girls as young as twelve years and under are on diets in order to make themselves thin.

Attempts to find biological bases for all of the above "disorders" are underway. I believe the greater part of the problem lies, not in our biology, but rather in our socio-cultural beliefs and practices. This is not to say that there may not be some biological determinants that predispose us to a scattering of these problems. Too often, we treat biology and environment as comprising mutually exclusive phenomena, ignoring the complex interplay between the many factors that produce human behaviour. This is why the biopsychosocial approach is a superior one, precisely because it understands the interconnectedness of these factors. If it were true that there was in fact a gene for eating disorders, this would not necessarily mean that there is nothing that can be done to prevent that gene from determining behaviour. The environment provides the impetus for genes to exert their action. Genes are a blueprint for the range of possibilities that exist to us. In a climate where women are valued for who we are and the contributions that we can make to humanity, where what we look like does not determine our worth, where our bodies are not used to sell products, it is doubtful that women who may have a predisposing gene for eating disorders will starve themselves to near death.[2] Biology is not destiny.

Toward a Feminist Psychology

So, what is to be done? Is it a completely hopeless situation? Is a feminist psychology conceivable? I believe it is. The first step should be a recognition that, while we debate the usefulness of labels and diagnostic categories, they are still being applied, without question, to women who are in pain. In the immediate present, questions of etiology are irrelevant to the women whose cases we argue. Many women need support in their attempts to cope with the distress that comes with living in a patriarchal society. Mental health practitioners should provide care and counselling to the best of their ability, taking each woman's life situation into account. But many other women need answers to the question of how we can build a more woman-positive praxis. Answers can only be forthcoming when we all acknowledge the continuum of experience and behaviour that exists between mental health and illness, along which we can all be situated at different times in our lives. I have tried to argue that much of what is labelled as pathological behaviour in women often amounts to behaviour that is prescribed of the stereotypical female role (dependent personality disorder, self-defeating personality disorder), or otherwise, normal psychic responses to pathological life situations (depression, multiple personality disorder, eating disorders). I have called this phenomenon pathologization of normalcy. It is my view and the view of other critics (Chesler, 1972; Miles, 1988; Russell, 1995; Ussher, 1991) that this phenomenon has specific political objectives that best serve the interests of the small group of White, straight, middle-class, Christian men who hold power in the West and wield it in the rest of the world. I now want to look at how we might integrate the insights of the past and the knowledge of the present to inform the praxis of the future.

Politicizing Psychology

As I have tried to show in this paper, psychology has colluded with and compounded our oppression. Kitzinger (1991) notes it is:

> ... harder to fight your oppression if you have been sold the idea that secretly you want it, that your raging hormones and your feminine "inner space" predispose you to submission; it is harder to build feminist alternatives if they have convinced you that you are sabotaging your own efforts at liberation, engineering your own failure, and that it is all your own fault for being insufficiently assertive, independent, and rational – in short for not being a man. (p. 50)

One of the first steps towards a feminist psychology is politicizing mainstream psychology. This means fighting battles on two fronts. On one front it means broadening the scope of psychological inquiry to include political discussions. Feminist psychologists and psychology in general must move to a location where it is both permitted and required that practitioners design and interpret research not simply in terms of scientific adequacy but perhaps, more importantly, the extent to which these validate the experiences of women and the extent to which they make a useful contribution to social transformation (Kitzinger, 1991). It is time to return to the vision of the early psychologists, but this time considering all of human experience. While I accept that psychology has the potential to reveal truths that could benefit the human population, I know that the theories and methods employed for the majority of psychological history are inadequate for that task.

On another front, politicizing psychology means using the tools of psychology – therapy, research – today, but never losing sight that the ultimate goal for tomorrow is social transformation. Using the analogy of a boxing match, Caplan (1992) cautions feminist therapists about the risk of becoming complicit in the oppression of women by giving them just enough support to go back into the ring and take more abuse. From my own work in a women's centre I know this to be a very real concern. I can identify with the frustration of seeing a woman in pain or distress and not being able to do anything more than offer her comfort, empathy, and support. Caplan also provides interesting food for thought for feminist therapists when she wonders whether, by doing therapy, we may inadvertently reinforce the idea that most of women's unhappiness comes from their inner selves. But what is the way out of this dilemma? Do we stop providing therapy when we know that so many women depend on the therapy hour as a much-needed reprieve from the madness?

Increased Activism

Both Caplan (1992) and Kitzinger (1991) suggest a way out of this rock-and-a-hard-place dilemma. According to Caplan, good feminist therapy should not be a substitute for transforming the world. She suggests that feminist therapists are in a unique position in that they have amassed a wealth of information about the systematic oppression of women and are therefore in a position to provide clues as to how that transformation could be made. Dominelli and McLeod (1989) also support this view that feminist therapy cannot be a substitute for collective political action by women. This principle is consistent with the Feminist Therapy Institute's, Feminist Therapy Code of Ethics (1987) which calls for feminist therapists to be committed to "political and social change that equalizes power among people" and "assume a proactive stance toward the eradication of oppression ... and work toward empowering women." Waterhouse (1993) provides a useful starting point with regard to bridging the gap between individual therapy and political action. For her, feminist therapy must do two things: help women deal with individually experienced pain which has its origin in the social, and enable the individual woman to see her experience as part of women's collective experience. In other words, the depathologizing of the individual must first be replaced with the problematizing of gender relations and an examination of the power relationships that inform those relationships. It is from an understanding of these that women can conceive of the need to act collectively. For many women, the therapeutic hour is the only forum from which this insight may come.

Democratization and Embodiment of Psychological Discourse

Sampson (1991; 1996) calls for a democratization of psychology and an embodiment of psychological discourse, which he sees as critical steps towards liberating psychology from the epistemological and methodological traps that have derailed its revolutionary potential in the past. I incorporate these into my own proposals for a feminist psychology because I see how they fit with fundamental principles of feminism as I understand them. I will explain. Sampson acknowledges that the process of democratization is already underway in psychology and other areas of inquiry. As we have already seen, the products of psychological inquiry (what he calls "outputs") have already been widely distributed to "the people." Sampson urges, however, that this process will only be over when the "inputs" of psychological inquiry are democratized, i.e., when a greater voice is given to "the people" who then have an input into the terms by which human knowledge, experience, and meaning are understood. This process necessarily involves giving people back their subjectivity, both in terms of their own experience and, literally, by seeing them as more than objects of our psychological studies. In this manner, Sampson suggests, they can be co-authors of our work. This view is consistent with the goals of feminist research practices which seek to give voice to those who have been silenced, represent difference, and celebrate diversity, start from personal experience by raising consciousness and working for social change, politicizing the personal (Reinharz, 1992).

Sampson (1996) also proposes what he calls an embodied psychological discourse. He criticizes psychology and other disciplines of the western tradition for their occularcentric bias; that is, their focus on phenomena that can be perceived visually. This, he argues, has produced a science that can only understand phenomena through observation and manipulation from outside. In order to know an object we must observe it from outside of it. Taken to its logical conclusion then, knowing and being are separate mutually exclusive activities. The mind and body relationship is severed. In psychology we have the example of the observer/psychologist observing the observed/object in a disembodied manner. Changing the language to call the observed a "participant" does nothing to alter the fundamental relationship with the observer/ psychologist.

My understanding of what Sampson calls for, is the establishment of a discourse in psychology that recognizes and applies the knowledge that all human phenomena and endeavours are embodied and are therefore socialized and signified, in particular social communities and particular social practices. Put simply, this goes back to the problem of contextualization. I have spent a great deal of time arguing here that women's behaviour patterns cannot be understood outside of the social contexts in which they have been socialized. In Sampsonian terms, this means that any attempt to unravel the complexities of women's behaviour patterns must account for how these have become embodied – that is, how they have come into being – and how they differ from men's behaviour patterns. To establish embodiment in psychological discourse is then to recognize these embodied qualities of all social practices, and that knowing and being are not always separate. One trope of feminist theory has attempted to address this situation by questioning the naturalness of the female (male) body, pointing instead to the ways in which it too is socially constructed. But what other characteristics should a feminist psychology possess?

Theorizing a Feminist Psychology

How can further psychological theorizing avoid the pitfalls that have produced a body of knowledge and associated practice that devalue the experiences of the majority? Let me recap.

As I have demonstrated, a shift in focus is crucial. Emphasis must be shifted away from the individual and placed on the larger social group. Individual behaviour cannot be fully understood when it is divorced form the context that produced and was produced by it. A feminist psychology should look like a fusion of sociology, psychology, and principles of feminism; social psychology does not go far enough. Perhaps this is what Koch (1993) means when he suggests a renaming of the discipline of psychology to "the psychological studies." Koch's main contention is that psychology cannot be a conceptually or theoretically coherent discipline. Rather it should be conceptualized as a collection of studies, some of which may count as science, but most of which do not.

Hollway (1991) contends, and I agree with her, that "[a] radical agenda for feminist psychology would politicize psychology with feminism rather than reduce feminism to psychology" (p. 30). It should be a discipline that seeks to understand the complex interplay between gender role socialization, the behavioural, cognitive and affective aspects of that socialization, and the effects of trauma or violence. Situated in a greater patriarchal culture where all forms of violence against women are the norm, a feminist psychology requires an analysis and contextualization of the effects of such violence on the psyche. It must fully understand and account for the role and meaning of interrelatedness and the social context, in women's lives. A feminist psychology must remain self-conscious of the psychological toll of sexism, racism, heterosexism, classism, sizeism, ableism, imperialism, on women's psychological development. But how might any of this be achieved?

A feminist psychology would make use of all the tools available to it. To this end it would employ various methodologies, recognizing that no one method is inherently less sexist than another, and that any method may be used in nonsexist ways (Peplau and Conrad,

1989). These must include narratives of women's lives, in their own voices. Reliance on a unimodal approach to psychological inquiry is no longer useful. Privileging one method over another is also useless. Multimodal approaches to the study of human experience should be encouraged as the way to more productive and comprehensive formulation of psychological theory.[3] If we take Koch's notion of psychological studies as a broad area of inquiry, it is clear that much of psychological study requires modes of inquiry and researcher training and background in areas other than the sciences.

A feminist psychology would avoid constructing a universal woman subject, since women do not make up a homogenous group. Instead, it would have as its point of departure, a recognition of the simultaneous sameness and difference of women's experience. A feminist psychology would place greater emphasis on the social group in which the individual finds herself, as the unit of analysis. Finally, a feminist psychology might begin to theorize and treat psychological distress as "problems in relations." Russell (1995) suggests focusing on relations instead of individuals and asking the following questions: How are relations structured within a particular social group? Which relations are harmful? To whom? For whose benefits? How can harmful relations be changed to promote human growth and fulfillment? This approach allows feminist psychologists to include men in their analyses, as men are integral parts of relational units and play extremely significant roles in many women's lives. It is crucial for feminist psychologists and other feminist scholars and activists to include in their analyses, the ways in which constructions of masculinity are harmful to women, as well as men.

Summary and Conclusion

As a solution to the madness, I have called for a more feminist psychology. What might this look like? I have suggested we begin by politicizing mainstream psychology and encouraging legitimate psychology inquiry to include political discourse. This would translate into, among other things, increased activism on the part of feminist therapists, who would recognize the need to bridge the gap between individual therapy and political action. Democratization and embodiment of psychological discourse would mean giving back subjectivity to the people who have been wounded by psychological discourse and having them become co-authors of psychological research. It would also mean recognizing and applying the knowledge that all human phenomena are context specific and, therefore, signified in particular communities and social contexts. This feminist psychology would employ multimodal approaches to the study of human experience and would avoid the temptation to construct a universal woman subject. Finally, this feminist psychology, applying all the strategies mentioned above, would begin to ask questions about pathological relations and situations, as opposed to asking questions about pathological individuals. In this process, it is crucial that traditional gender roles and unequal relations of power between and among groups of people, be held up to scrutiny, critique, and transformation.

Endnotes

1   While Freud himself must be held accountable for the misogyny behind his grand theories, it must be mentioned that much of what has been taken for psychoanalysis in this area, is not psychoanalysis in the strictest sense, since it was not expounded on by Freud himself, but by Helene Deutsch (1947) with Freud's blessing. For example, Freud himself never used the term "Electra complex" in his writings. This was a term coined by Helene Deutsch to refer to the female version of the Oedipus complex. She was also responsible for much of the early work on women's masochism. In fact her book *The psychology of women: A psychoanalytic interpretation* contains a chapter on "Feminine Masochism."

2   I first encountered the argument I make here in some earlier research on intelligence testing. In a study conducted by Sinnott, Dunn, and Dobzhansky, it was revealed that genetically identical Himalayan rabbits when reared in different environmental conditions, presented different observable characteristics (White body and Black extremities under natural conditions, and completely white bodies when reared in a warm cage). The idea here is that it is entirely possible for genetically identical individuals to display differences in observable traits that have high heritabilities. For more on this see Ronald J. Samuda, *Psychological testing of American minorities: Issues and consequences* (New York: Harper and Row, 1975).

3   The use of multiple methods in a single study has been referred to as "triangulation." I first came across this term in Shulamith Reinharz, *Feminist methods in social research* (New York: Oxford, 1992), p. 197. For more on this see Kevin Eckert's "Ethnographic Research on Aging," in Shulamith Reinharz and Graham Rowles, eds., *Qualitative gerontology* (New York: Springer, 1988), pp. 241–55.

References

Al-Issa, I. (1980). *The psychopathology of women*. Englewood Cliffs, N.J.: Prentice-Hall.

American Psychiatric Association. (1994). *Diagnostic and statistical manual of mental disorders, fourth edition*. Washington, D.C.

Barnes, M. and Maple, N. A. (1992). *Women and mental health: Challenging the stereotypes*. Birmingham, England: Venture.

Bem, S. L. (1993). Is there a place in psychology for a feminist analysis of the social context? *Feminism and Psychology 3*, 230–34.

Brown, L. S. and Ballou, M., eds. (1992). *Personality and psychopathology: Feminist reappraisals*. New York: Guilford.

Broverman, I. K., Broverman, D. M., Clarkson, F. E., Rosenkrantz, P. S., and Vogel, S. (1970). Sex role stereotypes and clinical judgments of mental health. *Journal of Consulting and Clinical Psychology 38*, 1–7.

Cannon, L. W. (1989). *Depression among women: Exploring the effects of race, class and gender.* Memphis: Centre for Research on Women, Memphis State University.

Caplan, P. J. (1987). The Psychiatric Association's failure to meet its own standards: The dangers of self-defeating personality disorder as a category. *Journal of Personality Disorders 1*, 178–82.

— (1991). How do they decide who is normal? The bizarre, but true, tale of the DSM process. *Canadian Psychology 32*, 162–70.

— (1992). Driving us crazy: How oppression damages women's mental health and what we can do about it. *Women and Therapy 12*(3), 5–28.

— (1992). Gender issues in the diagnosis of mental disorder. *Women and Therapy 12*(4), 71–82.

Caplan, P.J., & Gans, M. (1991). Is there Empirical Justification for the Category of "Self defeating personality disorder"? *Feminism and Psychology 1*(2), 263–78.

— (1991) DDPD: Consequences for the profession of psychology. *Canadian Psychology 32*(2), 136–38.

Caplan P. J. and Larkin, J. (1992). The gatekeeping process of the DSM. *Canadian Journal of Community Mental Health 11*, 17–28.

Chesler, P. (1972). *Women and madness.* New York: Doubleday.

Chodorow, N. J. (1989). *Feminism and psychoanalytic theory.* New Haven: Yale University.

Condor, S. (1991). Sexism in psychological research: A brief note. *Feminism and Psychology 3*, 430–34.

Deutsch, H. (1947). *The psychology of women: A psychoanalytic interpretation.* London: Research Books.

Dominelli L. and McLeod, E. (1989). *Feminist Social Work.* London: Macmillan.

Franks, V. and Rothblum, E. D. (1983). *The stereotyping of women: Its effects on mental health.* New York: Springer.

Hollway, W. (1991). The psychologization of feminism or the feminization of psychology? *Feminism and Psychology 1*, 29–37.

Kaplan, M. (1983). A woman's view of DSM-III. *American Psychologist 38*, 788–90.

Kitzinger, C. (1991). Politicizing psychology. *Feminism and Psychology 1*, 49–54.

Koch, S. (1993). "Psychology" or "the psychological studies"? *American Psychologist 48*, 902–4.

Larkin, J. & Caplan, P.J. (1992). The Gatekeeping process of the DSM. *Canadian Journal of Community Mental Health 2*(1), 17–27.

Lee, S., Chiu, H.F., Chen, C.N. (1989). Anorexia nervosa in Hong Kong: why not more in Chinese? *British Journal of Psychiatry 154*, 683–88.

Miles, A. (1988). *The neurotic woman: The role of gender in psychiatric illness.* New York: New York University.

Millon, T. (1967/1983). *Theories of personality and psychopathology.* New York: CBS College.

Nye, R. D. (1981). *Three psychologies: Perspectives from Freud, Skinner, and Rogers.* Monterey, CA: Brooks/Cole.

Parker, I., Georgaca, E., Harper, D., (1995). *Deconstructing pathology*. London: Sage.

Pantony, K. L. & Caplan P.J. (1991). Delusional Dominating Personality Disorder: a modest proposal for identifying the consequences of rigid masculine socialization. *Canadian Psychology 32*(2), 120–33.

Peplau, L. A. and Conrad, E. (1989). Beyond non-sexist research: The perils of feminist methods in psychology. *Psychology of Women Quarterly 13*, 379–400.

Perkins, R. E. (1991). Women with long-term mental health problems: Issues of power and powerlessness. *Feminism and Psychology 1*, 131–39.

Putnam, F. W., Guroff, J.J., Silberman, E.K., Barban, L., Post, R.M. (1986). The clinical phenomenology of multiple personality disorder: Review of 100 recent cases. *Journal of Clinical Psychiatry 47*, 285–93.

Reinharz, S. (1992). *Feminist Methods for Social Action Research*. New York: Oxford University.

Rosewater, L.B. (1987). A critical analysis of the proposed self-defeating personality disorder. *Journal of Personality Disorders 1*, 190–95.

Russell, D. (1995). *Women, madness and medicine*. Cambridge, MA: Polity.

Sampson, E. (1991). The democratization of psychology. *Theory and Psychology 1*, 275–98.

— (1996). Establishing embodiment in psychology. *Theory and Psychology 6*, 601–24.

Schaffer, K. F. (1980). *Sex-role issues in mental health*. Reading, MA: Addison-Wesley.

Spitzer, R. L., and Williams, J., eds. (1987). *Diagnostic and statistical manual of mental disorders* (3rd rev. ed.). Washington, DC: American Psychiatric Association.

Székely, E. (1988). *Never too thin*. Toronto: Women's Press.

Ussher, J. (1991). *Women's madness: Misogyny or mental illness?* Amherst, MA: University of Massachusetts.

Walker, L.E.A. (1987). Inadequacies of the Masochistic personality disorder diagnosis for women. *Journal of Personality Disorders 1*, 183–89.

Walkerdine, V. (1990). *School girl fictions*. London: Virago.

Waterhouse, R. (1993). 'Wild women don't have the blues': A feminist critique of person-centered' counselling and therapy. *Feminism and Psychology 3*, 55–71.

Wenegrat, B. (1995). *Illness and power: Women's mental disorders and the battle between the sexes*. New York: New York University.

Wiener, M and Marcus, D. (1993). A socio-cultural construction of "depression." In T. R. Sarbin and J. I. Kitsuse, eds. *Constructing the social* (pp. 213–31). London: Sage.

All Colours of the Rainbow: Recently Arrived Immigrant Women of Colour and HIV/AIDS in Canada

FARAH M. SHROFF

HIV/AIDS is the most politicized pathology in the modern world. It is shrouded within popular misconceptions, simple stereotypes that lightly veil the hatred for marginalized groups, and various unjusti-fied fears. Many marginalized groups have been blamed for and live with HIV/AIDS; gay men, Africans in the continent and within the diaspora, sex-trade workers, intravenous drug users, and others.

In this paper, I will focus on women of colour, a group of people living with AIDS (PLWAs) that rarely makes the media spotlight. However, approximately 90 per cent of HIV (Human Immuno Virus) positive[1] women live in the *south world*.[2] India contains a mushrooming HIV/AIDS epidemic that the world has heard very little about. "Even using a conservative estimate of infections, five million by the end of 1998 and doubling every three years, there will be a hundred million Indians infected by the year 2010 if not sooner."[3] This figure promises to be higher than the rest of the world combined in the next decades.

Indian women, like virtually all women of colour, will be getting HIV from their husbands. In some cases, a woman is aware that her husband engages in high-risk activities that jeopardize her health, but the pressure to reproduce or just to allow him to gain access to her body is so strong that she knowingly engages in unprotected intercourse with him. For other women, their husbands do not dis-close their high-risk behaviour or HIV+ status and the woman finds out that she is positive inadvertently – usually after she experiences unexplained health problems and gets them checked at a clinic.

DOUGLAS COLLEGE LIBRARY

Regardless, male power over women is largely responsible for the spread of the virus.

Canada and Immigrant Women

The vast majority of immigrants to Canada are generally young, well educated, and in good health. Data reveal that most immigrants probably contract the virus in Canada – they are not HIV+ upon arrival.

To illustrate the subtleties of the issues, I'm going to read a story of an immigrant woman of colour living with the virus. It illustrates the compromised legal rights of many dependent, immigrant women of colour, who are sponsored by their husbands and have few perceived and real ways of exercising their autonomy. It also illustrates the isolation that many women of colour experience due to language barriers, and the fact that abuse and violence often co-exist with HIV, serving to further isolate women. It is also a story of hope, of a woman piecing her life back together and gaining strength.

A SURVIVOR'S STORY [4]

> Nine years ago, my husband and I came to Canada. A few years later, and after a series of recurring infections, I was diagnosed with HIV. My doctor said he wanted to test my husband and daughter also; it was a terrible moment in an already shaky marriage.

> Things had been bad since we immigrated. My husband is a violent man, always blaming me for everything that goes wrong. When we learned that he was HIV+, things exploded. He accused me of giving him the virus, but I was not a drug user, I was a virgin when we married, and he is the only man I have ever had sex with. When I, in turn, accused him, he grew angry. He said that because I was much sicker than him, it must have been me that was infected first. My doctor said that I was more advanced in

my illness because my immune system is weaker: I have carried and cared for two children and there have been many physical and emotional demands on me. (I have accepted that I must now live with AIDS and no longer think about how I got infected, but my husband still continues to get tested at private clinics.)

When our doctor told us that we were both HIV+ but our daughter was negative, he also told us not to have any more children. Reluctantly, my husband used a condom, and soon after I obtained a prescription for birth control pills. Because I could speak very little English then, I do not know if the doctor told my husband to continue to wear a condom to prevent re-infection.

Unfortunately, I depended on my husband for everything. I have no family in Canada, and it was a long time before I could speak English. Things would have been different in my home country; my father and brothers would have stopped him from hitting me. But I cannot go back. I haven't enough money, my health is too poor, and my family has other problems. I do not want to be a burden. I write to them, but they do not know why I am sick.

My husband and I separated, and I stopped using the pill. We got back together again after he said he missed my daughter and me, and he acted so nice for a while. We had unprotected sex and I got pregnant. When he found out, he was furious. He accused me of trapping him and pressured me to have an abortion. But I could not kill this baby. My son is now fifteen months old, and tests still show that he is negative.

In the last three months things have changed. I have a good doctor and I go to see him without my husband. I have a kind and supportive AIDS worker. I wish I had met her earlier; without her I would not have had the courage to take control of my life. My children and I are moving to an apartment of our own with the aid of Family Benefits Allowance. The congregation of the church where I go is trying to raise enough money to bring my sister to Canada; if something happens to me, I want my sister to take care of my children.

I feel so relieved that I no longer have to depend on my husband, and I am happy that my children and I will finally have a peaceful home. I do not know how long I've got, but each day I take care of myself and my children, so that I can live with them for as long as possible.

Current Immigration Laws[5]

Canada's *Immigration Act* distinguishes between visitors,[6] immigrants, and refugees (1995).[7] Specific regulations apply to each of the categories, and various exceptions exist; it is not the purpose of this paper to outline in detail the legal aspects of immigration laws.

In general, all categories of people are subjected to the same entry criteria with respect to their medical status; that is, people who may be judged to fall within the following criteria may be deemed medically inadmissible to Canada:

a) The person constitutes a threat to public health or safety; OR
b) The person may cause excessive demands on health or social services.

Clearly, these criteria are subjectively defined, and are subjectively interpreted by visa or immigration officers. These officers, with a mere suspicion, may make a medical examination mandatory.

Most people seeking to enter Canada require a medical examination. While there is currently no mandatory HIV test as part of this examination, their HIV status could be determined in one of two ways by the medical officer who examines them. Firstly, the physician will ask if the person has ever tested positive for HIV or any other immune deficiency. Secondly, if the physician believes that it is clinically indicated, s/he can require HIV testing.

Immigration regulations afford physicians and immigration and visa officers an enormous amount of personal judgment. While this appears to be flexible and helpful in theory, the practice of this subjectivity allows deep-seated discriminatory attitudes on the part of these officials to be differentially applied to people seeking to enter Canada. Indeed, racism, sexism, heterosexism, and other forms of oppression, are routinely experienced by people seeking to enter the country.

HIV+ people are generally excluded from entering Canada because they will cause excessive demands on the public purse. Three legal cases to date have resulted in HIV+ people being admitted to the country on compassionate and humanitarian grounds, largely based on family reunification.

Clearly, this is not a huge number and most certainly shows that immigration is not a significant causal factor in the spread of HIV/AIDS in Canada.

Bill C-31

On September 20, 2000, newspapers reported that the Liberal government was planning to make changes to immigration laws: making HIV testing mandatory for all prospective immigrants and excluding those who tested positive as the "best public health option." As was just discussed, in practice, under the current law, most people seeking immigration to Canada have a good chance of being tested for HIV and being barred from entry if they test positive. This proposed change, Bill C-31, would make the regulations less focussed on individual people and their particular circumstances than on their disease classification. Similar to the current law, refugees and family-class, sponsored immigrants would be exempted.

The proposed change has raised the ire of most HIV/AIDS activists and they have many arguments against this proposed legislation. I'll list only a few. The opponents to the legislation note that testing specifically for HIV further labels and stigmatizes people living with HIV/AIDS and does not fit with Canada's reputation as a caring nation. They argue that many people living with HIV are healthy contributing members of society and it is unfair to rule them inadmissible on medical grounds. They argue that by testing for HIV, a slippery slope to ruling out people with other conditions is created, and it becomes difficult to know where to stop the sliding.

Rarely acknowledged in these arguments is the cost of health care services for people living in the advanced stages of HIV/AIDS. Research conducted in B.C., before the more costly anti-retroviral 'cocktails' became the standard treatment for HIV/AIDS showed that the last years of life for a PLWA costs approximately $150,000 per person.[8]

Because of the early election call, Bill C-31 has become dormant. We'll have to wait until after the election to see if the next government decides to take this up this kind of Bill again.

However, it is vital to examine the timing and the import of these proposed changes, regardless of whether they become law or not. Why did the Liberal government choose to make this announcement at a time when the Canadian Alliance Party appears to be making political advances nationally? Tax cuts for the rich; anti-immigrant laws; two-tiered medical care – all these things can be delivered by the Liberals too, and they're busily showing Canadians how quickly they can mimic Alliance policies. Bill C-31 is not based on facts but on perceptions of immigrants as vectors of disease.

POLICY ISSUES

We know that the vast majority of immigrants to this nation add to the youthful, productive, and healthful sectors of the population, and that they are a net economic and social addition to Canada. There is virtually no data to indicate that immigrants are the source of the Canadian HIV/AIDS pandemic. Bill C-31 feeds into anti-immigrant hysteria and AIDS phobia. Like many politically motivated legal changes, it is incumbent upon researchers and activists to struggle for immigration laws that are based on carefully collected data and analysis.

Recommendations that are specifically focussed on immigrant women of colour are more based in social and structural changes than on simple policies that can be passed by governments. Structural conditions under which immigrant women of colour, particularly those belonging to the working classes, live are based on globalized capitalist and racist patriarchal norms; these macroconditions graft themselves onto women's bodies and many illnesses and conditions result.

Women must have choices about who their partners are, about their decision to have intercourse with a particular person or not, about participating in a non-monogamous social order that only benefits men, about their desire to become pregnant and subsequently mothers, and many. many more such issues.

Specifically, learning about the body, pleasure, and sexuality, within the context of larger structural changes mentioned above, would help give women a language to discuss their own likes and dislikes. Having economic, social, and psychological situations that can allow women to say YES when it feels right and NO when it doesn't is a major benefit of these kinds of changes.

For women of colour around the world, HIV/AIDS is the medical result of various social oppressions. Since medical cures don't exist for HIV/AIDS and their related mortalities, social justice changes are the most potent promise as both prevention and *cure* for this deadly virus.

Endnotes

1. Please note that throughout this paper I will be citing data both for people living with AIDS and data for people who are HIV+. These data are often confused with each other; this is a serious mistake. People who have been diagnosed with AIDS are much more easily counted than those who are seropositive (HIV+), because in many cases testing is voluntary, and not all HIV+ want to find out, or for other reasons do not get tested.

2. UNAIDS 1999; AIDS Five Years Since ICPD: Emerging issues and challenges for Women, Young People, and Infants. UNAIDS Discussion Document. 20 Avenue Appia, 1211 Geneva 27, Switzerland.

3. Rajan Gupta, "The HIV/AIDS Pandemic in India is Real," from AIDS Crisis in India website http://t8 web.lanl.gov/people/rajan/AIDS-india/MYWORK/summary.3.99.html

4. From "Double Jeopardy: Women, Violence and HIV," vis-à-vis, Canadian Council on Social Development, http://www.hc-sc.gc.ca/hppb/familyviolence/html/vol13n3e/vol13n3e.htm

5. Much of the information in the sections pertaining to Immigration Regulations and the Law is gleaned from "HIV/AIDS and Immigration: A Draft Discussion Paper," by Alana Klein for the Canadian HIV/AIDS Legal Network 2000.

6. Not all visitors are required to take a medical examination. Immigration regulations require those of a "prescribed class" to take a medical examination. They are: 1. Visitors in particular occupations where the protection of the public is essential; 2. Persons who wish to remain in Canada for longer than 6 months; and 3. Visitors who have recently resided in a country where the incidence of communicable disease is higher than in Canada (Immigration Regulations, SOR/78-172, s21).

7. A visitor is someone who enters Canada for temporary purposes, such as tourism, to study at a Canadian educational institution, short-term workers. An immigrant is someone who seeks to make Canada their permanent residence. A convention refuge is someone who is: a) outside their country of nationality or former habitual residence, and b) has a well-founded fear of persecution due to their race, religion, nationality, membership in a particular social group, or political opinion, and c) are unable or, owing to that fear, unwilling to return to their country of origin. Refugees are divided into two categories, each of which is governed differently: those seeking entry from within Canada or at the border, and those applying from abroad for settlement in Canada (Donald Galloway, *Immigration Law* (Concord, ON: Irwin Law, 1997)).

8. Robin Handvelt (personal communication, 2000). Associate Professor, Department of Health Care and Epidemiology, UBC.

A Model of Women Services in the HIV Epidemic

TALATA REEVES

"The deep truth is that our human suffering need not be an obstacle to the joy and peace we so desire, but can become, instead the means to it." – Henri J.M. Nouwen, *Life of the Beloved: Spiritual Living in a Secular World* (New York: Crossroad Publishing, 1991), p. 7.

The purpose of this article is to share some of what we have learnt about working with women and families in the HIV epidemic in the United States, specifically in New York City. Our hope is that some of the information and ideas discussed will be useful to other organizations and individuals providing HIV prevention and care services for women and families.

Founded in 1981 by volunteers, Gay Men's Health Crisis, Inc. (GMHC) is the oldest non-profit (NGO) HIV/AIDS service provider in the world. Our threefold mission is "to reduce the spread of HIV disease; to help people with HIV maintain and improve their health and independence; and to keep the prevention, treatment, and cure of HIV an urgent national and local priority." In 1991, the agency began the Child Life Program to serve women and families affected by HIV/AIDS. Prior to 1996, much of the work in Child Life focused on helping families through the death and dying process. In the HIV treatment era, the Child Life program addresses the growing needs of parents and families *living* with HIV. In 1992, GMHC expanded its services for women by establishing the Lesbian AIDS Project (LAP). Today, LAP continues its threefold mission: "to support lesbians living with HIV/AIDS, to provide HIV prevention information and education to lesbians and women who have sex with women (WSW), and to advocate for more research and education about woman to woman HIV transmission." In December 1996, GMHC continued to expand its efforts to meet the critical population shifts in the epidemic in New York City by establishing the Women and Family Services Department (WFS). In 1997, WFS began a new program initiative, Women in Action (WIA), targeting sex workers, injection drug users, undocumented immigrant women and others not in care, and women in all stages of substance use and recovery. WIA supports women to achieve psychosocial stabilization to access HIV care and stay in treatment.

The mission of WFS is to provide culturally competent outreach, education, early intervention, access to care and support for women and families at risk for or living with HIV/AIDS. WFS provides a wide range of services including group and individual counselling, family social support, substance use counselling, nutritional counselling, food pantry, emergency food services, acupuncture, complementary therapies, crisis intervention and referrals. WFS clients have immediate access to other GMHC services, such as treatment education, meals, case management, and legal services. Through its playroom, WFS provides childsitting support for women and all parents receiving services from the agency. Childsitting or childcare is an essential component to ensuring that women are able to access the needed services while their children are being cared for in a nurturing and child-friendly environment. All of these services provide psychosocial stabilization of women living with HIV/AIDS, access to treatment, and maintenance in care.

WFS provides individual and group level HIV prevention interventions targeting poor women, women of colour, and other women at high risk for HIV infection (i.e., sex workers and substance users). One-on-one interventions take place on-site and at a variety of outreach venues (health fairs, bars, clubs, other agencies, and street outreach). We distribute safer sex kits and educational materials at all outreach events. The majority of our safer sex kits and written materials are designed for specific populations of women.

Our group level interventions include workshops, forums, conferences, and other educational initiatives that reach both women living with HIV/AIDS, women at risk for HIV infection, and service providers.

Women Services in a Gay Organization

The provision of women services in a gay organization has been perceived as highly unorthodox. Fundamental questions as to why a gay organization would provide women services, and equally important, why would women seek services in a gay organization are often asked. For GMHC, the inception on HIV services for women was a natural outcome of its mission to serve the emerging populations in the epidemic. For the last ten out of its twenty years of service in the epidemic, GMHC has been serving women and families through dedicated programs. In that time, we have discovered some distinct advantages to providing women and family services in this context.

Anonymity and Safety

Twenty years into the HIV/AIDS pandemic, the stigma of living with HIV continues to be very real. As a result, many women seek HIV services outside their communities rather than risk disclosure of their HIV status. Through GMHC, women have access to HIV care while ensuring anonymity of their HIV status in their communities. Approximately 66 per cent of women living with HIV and AIDS in the United States have histories of violence (including rape) and 30 to 40 per cent report childhood sex abuse (Hader, Smith, Moore, Holmberg, 2001). Our women clients report feeling "safe" here because they experience significantly less exposure to sexual advances. For them, receiving services among primarily gay rather than straight men provides them with "sexual safety." Additionally, this setting provides some freedom from socialized competition for male attention, which in turn creates the space for women to focus on themselves and engage in self-directed decision-making.

One-Stop Shopping and Quality of Care

As the first AIDS service organization in the United States, GMHC has developed considerable expertise in working with the issues of HIV risk and care in the epidemic. This expertise translates into a high standard of care for people living with HIV (PLWH) and people living with AIDS (PLWA). WFS clients benefit from the expertise and the breadth of GMHC's services. Additionally, GMHC's "one-stop shopping" model is supportive and user-friendly for women. On a typical day, a woman can leave her child in the playroom, go to a women's group, see her counsellor, have lunch in the meals program, see a lawyer or a treatment education counsellor, get support around her HIV benefits, and then pick up her child before going home. Providing critical HIV services in one location ensures access to HIV care for women who have multiple care-taking responsibilities that often prevent them from receiving services.

Transformation and Self-Reflection

Our philosophy of HIV services is based on the premise that HIV work is more than the delivery of tangible or concrete services to women. HIV is a disease that has its root causes in both social and personal "dis-ease." HIV can be understood as the physical manifestation of the deeper social problems that put women at risk for transmission. All forms of gender bias, the under-education and mis-education of young girls, the feminization of poverty, reproductive control, homophobia, sexual oppression, and violence, to name a few, are at the source of women's risk of HIV infection. The degree to which women have control over their bodies and their lives is directly proportional to their exposure and vulnerability to HIV infection. HIV risk is rooted in how women internalize this oppression and how it is manifested in lives of desperation and despair. HIV is as much about how women are valued in their cultures as it is about the mechanics of transmission.

Self-exploration is a critical component of HIV prevention and is a rare commodity in women's lives. In most cases, it is non-existent for poor women who lack the resources, the time, and the familial support to focus on their own needs. Concrete services are critical because women are not going to be able to do transformational work if they are hungry or if they are worried about who is watching their children. By meeting their life sustaining needs, women have the freedom to engage in transformational work. Transformational work transcends the skills-based approach to behaviour change. It has a psychological intervention component that addresses issues such as, dependency and codependency, trauma, self-esteem, self-image, decision-making, and personal autonomy. Among women, transformational work can have a significant impact in their health and well-being. For example, in the general population, the greater incidence of depression among women may be linked to how women value themselves and their lives in the context of cultural, religious, and other forms of repression and oppression. Among HIV-positive women, 60 per cent report depressive symptoms consistent with the degree of psychological stress that make up their lives (Hader et al., 2001). A new longitudinal study of HIV disease progression in women reconfirms the link to and the adverse effects of depression among HIV positive women with chronic depressive symptoms who are "two times more likely to die compared with those with limited or no depressive symptoms" (Ickovics et al., 2001). For women, the goal of transformational work is to understand the issues for HIV risk and care from personal and social perspectives. Transformational work builds self-esteem, fosters autonomy and self-advocacy, and is a critical component in facilitating sustainable changes in the patterns of thinking and the behaviours that perpetuate risk for HIV infection or that diminish the quality of the lives of women living with HIV and AIDS.

There are three primary approaches to our model of services: 1) harm reduction model, 2) peer model, and 3) whole woman/whole community model. The first two models are well-established approaches in the fields of the social and behavioural sciences. The third approach grew out of our experience of working with different populations of women in this setting. Our model is organic in nature and has evolved over the last ten years of targeting and working with women and families in the epidemic. This model is still being rede-fined by new information about HIV risk and the specific care needs for women and families impacted by HIV disease.

The Harm Reduction Model

The primary clinical approach of all GMHC services, including women services, is known as the Harm Reduction Model. This approach offers an alternative to the moral and disease models for changing behaviour. Harm reduction focuses on the consequences or the effects of drug use or a high-risk behaviour in the individual's life (Marlatt, 1996). In this model, the goal is to reduce or eliminate the harmful consequences of a particular behaviour or behaviours. "Harm reduction is not anti-abstinence. Harmful effects of unsafe drug use or sexual activity can be placed along a continuum, much like the span of temperature on a thermometer. When things get too hot or too dangerous, harm reduction promotes 'turning down the heat' to a more temperate level. This gradual 'step-down' approach encourages individuals with excessive or high-risk behaviour to take it "one step at a time" to reduce the harmful consequences of their behaviour" (Marlatt, 1996).

NON-LINEAR, COMPLEX, AND MULTI-LAYERED

The research supporting this model identifies five stages of change: pre-contemplation, contemplation, planning and preparation, action, and maintenance (Prochaska et al., 1992). In changing behaviours, getting from point *A* to point *B* is rarely a straight line. For the major-ity of individuals this process in non-linear. Behavioural change is complex and multi-layered, as it is imbedded in life histories with complexities such as trauma (i.e., rape, incest, and domestic violence). Depending on the complexity of her issues, a woman may be in several different stages of change at the same time. For exam-ple, she may be in the *contemplation stage* around her substance use, meaning she is aware that she has a problem and she is considering what to do about it. On the other hand, this same woman may be in the *action stage* around her HIV care; that is, she has made the necessary changes in her behaviour and environment to meet her care goals.

EASY ACCESS

To support easy access to services, multiple *ports of entry* are necessary. These ports of entry have different thresholds or intensities. Our low threshold ports of entry provide anonymous and drop-in services. Ports that provide high threshold services require confidential information and tend to be more structured around time and participation. For example, earpoint acupuncture is an anonymous (requiring minimal identifying information and no intake), drop-in (does not require an appointment) service and therefore considered to be a low threshold port of entry. Additionally, acupuncture is considered low threshold because it is primarily a non-verbal and non-threatening intervention that supports the mind-body-spirit connection. For some individuals, just getting to the program requires major behavioural change, and for those individuals low threshold services are critical. Conversely, services such as long-term therapy are considered high threshold or high intensity. To successfully engage in these services, individuals need to have greater psychosocial stabilization. The majority of our clients initially require low threshold or intensity services.

STRENGTH-BASED APPROACH

By the time women reach us, they have had many experiences of failure around drug use and changing other high-risk behaviours. Additionally, they present with low self-esteem and experience themselves as being unable to change or not worthy of change. Often, they do not see themselves as being capable of change or having experienced any success towards change. We utilize a strength-based approach to working with changing behaviours. The focus is on the glass being *half-full* rather than *half-empty*. One meets the individual where s/he is in the change process, rather than where s/he should be or needs to be. This approach identifies areas of success or strengths as the starting point. This partial success is the foundation upon which a woman can continue movement towards her goals.

For many women, this is a paradigm shift from the *all or nothing* approach to changing behaviour, to an appreciation of the innumerable small successes that make up changing a behaviour. Permanent behavioural change is a long process rich with set backs or relapses which are always opportunities for furthering growth.

The recognition of success in these small steps builds the self-confidence necessary to achieve goals in behavioural change.

In our experience, the harm reduction model is a very powerful approach for working with women. In this model, women participate as full partners in their care and decision-making rather than carrying out someone else's idea of what is best for them. Additionally, access to multiple thresholds of services supports the complexity of women's lives in their process of change. For example, consistently missing critical appointments may be evidence of the myriad issues and/or barriers faced by a woman. Perhaps she does not have reliable childcare, transportation, a substance use problem or a more involved emotional problem, or she may feel or believe that she cannot meet an expectation, or all the above. Providing drop-in services for a woman with these challenges increases her access to critical services. As she develops confidence, and as the other con-crete care needs are met, such as transportation support and childcare, she will be able to tolerate more intensive services for which she will need to be able to keep appointments. Multiple thresholds support incremental change and success; an essential component of sustainable behavioural change.

The Peer Model

For the last thirty years, the peer model has been proven an effective approach for supporting behavioural change (Tindall, 1995). Today, the model is used to address a wide range of societal problems, including poor academic achievement, drug and alcohol use, smoking, teenage pregnancy, suicide, low self-esteem, eating disorders, violence in communities, and HIV and AIDS. The proliferation of this model attests to its success and demonstrates the primacy of the peer relationship in achieving and sustaining behavioural change.

In WFS, peers are part of a multidisciplinary team that consists of professionals (formally trained staff), paraprofessionals (trained non-professionals or peers), and volunteers. The convergence of skills and experiences on the team enhances our ability to reach our target communities more effectively and provide women and families with a greater variety of interventions to support their goals. Peers are fully involved in the development, implementation, and evaluation of ongoing and new program initiatives. WFS peers provide support services to women living with HIV and AIDS or at risk of HIV infection, including co-facilitating psycho-educational groups, crisis intervention, referrals, outreach, events planning, childsitting, and social support. Although the majority of peers come with little or no formal work experience, they all come with rich life experiences. Some peers have successful employment histories that were interrupted as a result of their HIV disease. For all the peers, the program is a *return to work* bridge. Through educational opportunities, peers discover new talents and transfer some of their survival skills from the home, street corner, or prison to their current roles. During their tenure in the program, peers participate in specific training related to their work (e.g., basic counselling skills, both group and individual, and outreach), and receive support as they explore their employment and career options.

The WFS peers do more than learn new skills and deliver services. Our peers are women living with HIV and AIDS, women of colour, women with economic challenges, women with histories of incarceration, women in recovery, and women who are the primary care givers to young children and other generations in their families. Although HIV treatment prolongs life, the complexity of the regimens, the toxicity of the drugs, and the other side effects, present significant challenges for adherence. In addition to managing a life-threatening disease, their family responsibilities, and delivering services, our peers are engaged in the same transformational process as other women in the program. As learners and leaders, peers work toward conscious personal growth and integrated wholeness in order to sustain new attitudes and behaviours. To this end, peer educators participate in their own psychosocial and emotional support groups where they have the opportunity to integrate the professional and personal aspects of their experience.

As women living with HIV and AIDS, peers are powerful role models. They have a greater ability to influence at-risk women about the importance of staying HIV-negative. Their life transforming victories, achieved in spite of their disease, are compelling testimonies to the human spirit. Through the example of their lives, compassion, and empathy, peers make the intangible tangible and place the possibility of *something better than one's current reality* well within reach. They teach us all that life goes on after an HIV diagnosis. And that life can be richer, deeper, and have a greater impact than before. Indeed, the impact of their lives far exceeds the staff and clients in the programs. Like ripples on the water, through their courageous examples, peers transform their families and communities.

The peer model elevates women's wisdom and their lives because it supports and encourages the transfer of women's life experiences and skills to better serve their personal goals. In a shared learning context, women value their own and each others knowledge, develop new skills, and gain support for meeting the challenges of staying HIV negative or living with HIV/AIDS. Additionally, the peer model provides women with opportunities to give back to their community while being supported in a community of women with similar goals, aspirations, and experiences. Through participation in the peer program, women reconstitute and gain autonomy over their lives, build self-esteem, reduce HIV transmission, and increase their adherence in HIV care.

The Whole Woman/Whole Community Model

This approach for serving women in the epidemic is indigenous to WFS. We work in an environment where all women are welcome and feel at home, regardless of their sexual orientation, sexual behaviour, ethnicity, whether or not they have children, and the myriad other differences that define their lives. From daughter, lover, wife, mother, substance user, lesbian, heterosexual, to sister, friend, and so forth, women identify in many ways and fill many roles in their families and cultures. However, women are more than the roles and identities that they choose or that are forced upon them in their communities. Mothers are not *only* mothers and lesbians are not *only* women who partner with women. Additionally, one's identity as mother or lesbian changes over time. While there is a great deal of strength within our identities, moving beyond the confines of identity is far more reflective of its dynamic nature.

Many programs compartmentalize women's lives. These types of programs perpetuate and reinforce the fractured and disconnected experiences that are often at the root of the problems for which women seek help. Consequently, these programs force women to choose one identity or role in order to receive services. For example, a woman may receive services as a mother, but if she is a lesbian mother only one aspect of her identity may be dealt with in that setting. Nowhere is this compartmentalization more apparent than among heterosexual women and lesbians. One rarely finds women's programs that openly encourage participation of lesbians and bisexual women. Although lesbian and bisexual women are present in these programs, this aspect of their identity is usually not acknowledged and nurtured. It is as if in these settings, *womanhood* is defined by the gender of one's partner. This compartmentalized approach perpetuates the oppression of lesbian and bisexual women in the very contexts where they should feel safe, that is, among other women. Additionally, this approach does not reflect what we know about the complex and contradictory expressions of sexual identity and sexual behaviour.

We know that sexual identity and sexual behaviour are not necessarily static or congruent in the human experience. Cultural and religious traditions, internalized and societal homophobia, and a number of other factors influence the diverse spectrum of sexual behaviour and sexual identity. Some women who identify as heterosexual have sex with and partnerships with other women. Conversely, some women who identify as lesbians have sex with and partnerships with men. To adopt behaviours that reduce a woman's risk for HIV transmission, a non-judgmental environment where she can freely and openly explore the connections between behaviour, identity, and HIV risk is essential. To this end, we welcome the *whole woman*, including the configurations and expressions of her sexuality. We encourage her process of refining, redefining and/or integrating her sexual identity and behaviour in light of her risk for HIV infection.

HIV is a family disease. As the primary care givers in most family systems, when mom has HIV the whole family is affected. Partners, lovers, and spouses of women living with HIV/AIDS experience additional relational stress and familial responsibilities as a result of their partner's condition. HIV depletes the physical, emotional, and financial resources of individuals and families. All family members experience the social stigma of living with HIV at varying degrees. Fears of discrimination and of being ostracized from the community determine the extent to which families disclose their HIV status. Consequently, in multi-level HIV serostatus families (i.e., families with HIV-positive and HIV-negative members) there exist multi-levels of HIV disclosure. One child may know the parent's HIV status and the other child or children may not. The energy and effort placed into maintaining these levels of secrecy place tremendous psychological stress on families.

To support sustainable life changes, the woman's family or network of support has to be engaged at some level. In WFS, the definition of family is determined by the woman herself and may include or exclude member of her biological family. For many women, their family or network of support is the source of their greatest strengths and simultaneously the source of their greatest challenges. Her support system is not tangential to the healing process, but is the context in which healing and wholeness takes place. Strengthening families and networks of support increase the potential for success in reducing high-risk behaviours and managing HIV care. Additionally, working with families provides opportunities to impact the next generation. In most cases, the children in these families face some of the same risk factors as their parents (i.e., substance use). Many of these children have already been negatively impacted by the consequences of their parent's high-risk behaviours (e.g., substance use and incarceration). Additionally, they face all the challenges of growing up in a twenty-first century urban setting *and* living with HIV in the family. By working with the whole family, the potential exists to break the cycle and the devastation of HIV in next generation.

Conclusion

Today HIV/AIDS is in every country around the world. There were 5.3 million new HIV infections at the end of the year 2000 according to the UNAIDS. Of this number 2.2 million were women and 600,000 were children under the age of fifteen. Of the 36.1 million people living with HIV and AIDS today, 16.4 million are women and 1.4 million are children under fifteen years old. Only a small fraction of these individuals, primarily in industrialized countries, are being served in the pandemic. Already, service providers are overwhelmed by the immediate needs of people impacted by this pandemic. Reflection, a primary component of any discipline, is at best relegated to the periphery of the work. Equally significant, there are few opportunities for providers to share what they have learned about HIV prevention and providing compassionate care for people living with HIV/AIDS. We enhance our work by valuing reflection and shared learning as one of the ways in which we marshal our intellectual powers and experiences to meet the challenges of the pandemic. In this sense, the process of writing this article has been a gift for me and I hope that it has been both challenging and enlightening for the reader.

References

Hader, Shannon L., Smith, Dawn K., Moore, Janet S., Holmberg, Scott D. (2001). HIV infection in women in the United States. *Journal of the American Medical Association (JAMA)* 285(9), 1190.

Ickovics, Jeanette R., Hamburger, Merle E., Vlahov, David, Schoenbaum, Ellie E., Schuman, Paula, Boland, Robert J., & Moore, Janet. (2001). Mortality, CD4 cell count decline, and depressive symptoms among HIV-seropositive women. *Journal of the American Medical Association (JAMA)* 285(11), 1472.

Marlatt, G. A. (1996). Harm reduction: Come as you are. *Addictive Behaviors 21* (6), 779–88.

Prochaska, James O., DiClemente Carlo C., Norcross, John C. (1992). In search of how people change. *American Psychologist* (September): 1102–12.

Tindall, Judith A. (1995). *Peer programs: An in-depth look at peer helping.* Taylor and Francis Group, 51.

UNAIDS. (2000). Update on the HIV epidemic, December.

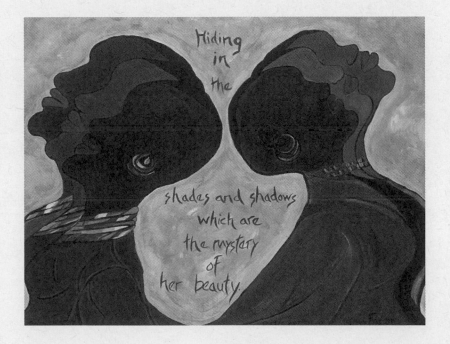

Healing Warrior Marks: Battling Stress

CRYSTAL E. WILKINSON

I had tried for years, but no amount of bubble baths, peaceful medi-tation, Iyanla Vanzant books, or Oprah segments could remove the superwoman 's' that seemed to be permanently tattooed in the centre of my chest above my breasts like a war scar. I don't even know when it appeared. It wasn't something I asked for. It just appeared. Maybe it began when I became a mother at seventeen as a second semester freshman in college, or later when I split from my children's father for good and declared "I wouldn't ever need anybody for nothing." Perhaps it was even earlier when I was a little brown girl with long spindly legs growing up in rural Kentucky and saw my Aunt Lovester and my Granny Christine doing it all and not getting or asking for help. I remember admiring their strength and vowing to be just like them when I grew up. Why did I embrace superwomanhood as though it was something I was supposed to do? Why have I walked around wearing it like a crown all these years? Proud of my *I-don't-need-nobody-for-nothin'* mantra. I can do it all! Or so I thought.

Last year, after a series of undiagnosed symptoms – heart palpi-tations, a flushing feeling, general nervousness, headaches, nausea, and not being able to sleep – my family physician called me into her office and handed me a prescription for antidepressant/anti-anxiety medication. I think you are having anxiety attacks, she said. I argued with her to the bitter end, declaring that I had been on my own since I was sixteen years old and hadn't had a panic attack ever in my life. "Tell me about your life," she said with that voice that we often reserve for our children. Taking her challenge on, knowing that I, above all people, had everything under control. I began to unfold with a vengeance, hell-bent on telling her off.

> I have three children: a twenty-year-old son (who at the time didn't have a job or plans to attend college); twin girls (in the height of puberty); I am an administrator for a non-profit organization (the kind of job that you can never leave completely once you leave); my book will be published soon (my publisher was in London, England and I was trying to tie up the loose ends via internet and express mail and everything had to be done ASAP, and simultaneously trying to plan a three-week summer creative writing program for high school students); my grandparents, who raised me, died over the last five years (leaving me with the greatest loss I have experienced to date); I am on six different community boards and committees (all tugging and pulling, but I was trying to "give back"); I'm at odds with various members of my family (a lot of suppressed anger); I am always financially strapped (mainly because of my children's fathers who won't pay and who have never paid child support).

Mind you, I am trying to tell her the surface information, and to answer only the questions she asks. The deeper information (in the parentheses) was held inside my heart, body, and soul like a hot secret that was searing through my body and mind, threatening spontaneous combustion. Before I could go any further, my doctor stopped me and began laughing. Not at me but with me, she would later explain. "Are you hearing yourself?" she asked.

The rest of the appointment was a blur. I remember seeing her face smiling at times, her eyebrows arching and her head shaking in disbelief at others. I nodded my head up and down, yes, as she talked, but I don't recall more than that. I was devastated and crying by the end of our appointment. Me, the superwoman, having *panic* attacks. I was thinking, I have done this, and accomplished this, and made my way through that, and now, this little white woman (she is only four feet nine) is telling me that I am having panic attacks. I must admit that I shrugged it off as white folks' rubbish for the first few weeks. I put it all out of my mind, at least on the forefront. But I was reminded every time I ran across the prescription slip in my purse, or every time I had another one of my *spells* as I came to call them (dizziness, heart racing, nausea, etc.). I kept reassuring myself that maybe it was high blood pressure or diabetes. Not that I wanted it to be those things, but those were family illnesses passed down from generation to generation. I was expecting diabetes, even though I watched my diet. My grandfather had it, my mother, my grandmother, my father. All of my aunts. My cousins. Even hypertension felt familial in some way, but not something that was in my head or stress related. Black women weren't supposed to have those kind of things. Or at least that is what I thought. So I continued to try and self diagnose. I sneaked into urgent treatment centres, health fairs, and even tried the health department. I wasn't ready to fight my insurance company for a second opinion and I wasn't ready to face my doctor. Each time I got my blood pressure or my blood sugar checked it was normal. I know it sounds silly but I was really willing to take a familiar illness over anything that had to do with my brain or stress. Life is life, I thought. There is no cure for life.

I finally went back to my doctor. Still not ready to give up, I asked her for a battery of specialists. She agreed and wanted to make sure she hadn't missed anything. She sent me to a neurologist, a gastrologist, a gynaecologist, and approved an array of heart, blood, and intestinal tests. Nothing. I went home scared and still not willing to face anxiety as a diagnosis. I began my own research on the Internet, spending a large portion of my work day and then staying up nights at home on the computer, searching every health-related dot com I could find. Finally, I, self-proclaimed Dr. Wilkinson, decided that perhaps it was hormonal, after all I had even had surgery to remove cysts on my ovaries that same year. The doctor said that perhaps I was premenopausal and prescribed estrogen. So that's it. I had finally found a satisfactory blame. At 37, I found myself in conversations with my fifty- and sixty-year-old counterparts about hot flashes, the values of soy, and the way we "used to be." But the symptoms didn't stop. I was still having dizzy moments and feelings of anxiety. I continued the hormone therapy for a year, just because I still didn't want to face the fact that it could be my lack of super-human strength to cope with my overstressed life that could be the source of my symptoms.

As someone who had been a vegetarian for years – and high on organic and natural foods – I finally came to the conclusion that pumping estrogen made from horse urine was as unhealthy as whatever was causing the symptoms. I took myself off the estrogen-replacement therapy and, after time had passed, had my hormones tested. The tests came back normal.

With a whoosh a year passed with my neck and shoulders always in such knots that I was in pain most of the time; headaches; being so stressed that if one more thing was piled on, I was sure my head would explode. I had also gained a dangerously high amount of weight. At the peak of it all, during stressful times at work, I could not breathe. I would lock myself in a stall in the bathroom and try to regain my breath by taking those long cleansing breaths I had learned in meditation classes, before heading out to teach that next class or to that next meeting. At home, I would be so wound up that I came into the door from work, stripping off my clothes and head-ing for the bed, where I would lay for hours until I could function. It became later and later into the evening before I could cook, clean, and do the other things that I had to do.

Meanwhile, I was still saying "yes" to boards, committees, public speaking engagements for the book, teaching workshops, friends in need, the newspaper carrier, strangers in the supermarket, my chil-dren, relatives who I knew hated me, my son's father (who I let move in with us when he fell upon hard times), and on and on. When one of my friends asked me what I had done for myself lately, I couldn't think of one thing.

Just like I couldn't remember when my superwoman scar had began to tear into my flesh, I can't now remember when I decided enough was enough, but I'm glad that I had the sense to begin to heal. I now know that perhaps if I had taken my doctor's advice and took the medication perhaps I would have felt better sooner. Medications have their purpose. I know that medication can be an integral part of healing from any kind of illness, but I also know that as someone who prides herself on being somewhat of a naturalist, I couldn't allow my stress to be band-aided by medication alone. It was up to me to begin my own healing journey. Once my mind was made up, I took all my superhuman strength (I can laugh about that now) and turned some of it toward myself. First, I added the word NO to my vocabulary. I sent out a flurry of e-mail and snail mail letters that began, "It is with great regret that I must resign from ..." and I did have *regret*. I think that I am addicted to stress. I really miss not doing something with every minute of my time. I think I have done it for so long that I feel like I'm being lazy when I'm not committed to someone else's interests. The other part of it was guilt about not taking care of someone else's needs first. As black women, we've been brought up that way. Just like we had training bras. I think we all received our miniature superwoman-in-training 's' in girlhood. I still have stressful days and all of my symptoms haven't totally subsided, but I am on a path to expel my own superwomanhood. I take one day a week and declare it MY day when everything that is done that day has to be beneficial to ME and ME only. Sometimes this involves being with other people. Sometimes it involves being alone. The hardest part of all this is not feeling selfish about doing something for me. I have also managed to make my diet changes, and going to the gym four times a week is a priority which in itself has alleviated almost all the symptoms.

It's still hard to quiet the mythological black woman/hero/doer-of-everything-for-everybody who got me where I am, but it's also refreshing to know that there is a vulnerable, strong sister who HAS to be taken care of under my warrior marks.

Taking Care

CRYSTAL E. WILKINSON

(For Granny Christine)

You nurtured me, embraced me in warm, soft hugs. You were not the one who gave me birth, but I was your sugar baby. It was you who blew dust from my eyes, nursed my fevers, kissed my bruises, and encouraged my dreams.

You were married at fourteen, cleaned houses for white folks, and still managed to raise seven children plus me, and attended Grand Daddy's every need. You were always somebody's something. I never really remember you taking care of yourself.

Maybe that's why you insisted that I *take care* every time we parted. Maybe that is why you pulled me close and whispered "Girl, if you don't take care of *you*, ain't gonna be nobody to do it." You told me to learn to take care of *me*. You said every woman should.

Whenever life got too hard, it was to you I ran. You always insisted that I put my feet up. You would cook biscuits and blackberries or whatever I wanted. You would tell me not to worry about the kids, to just rest. Only with you could I stop being the strong black woman and just be. You would look into the tiredness in my eyes, beyond the throbbing headache and tell me that I wouldn't be any good to anybody dead. That *taking care* was essential.

When you died, I didn't know what to do. Even when I thought I was coping, I would catch myself all clenched up tight as a fist, blood pressure rising, head hurting, suffering from superwoman blues. I was always working two jobs, taking care of three children alone, being the lean-on-me for all my friends. Not shedding a tear toward nobody for nothing. I wanted and needed you. I thought your arms were my only solstice.

You have been gone for some time and still, "Girl, you got to take care of yourself," echoes like thunder at those precise moments when I have had enough.

I am on the edge of understanding, on the edge of *taking care* like you said. I am slowly learning, growing toward balance.

Now, when I run, it is to my house, where I plan these long, leisurely dates with my strong-sister self. I get a baby sitter for the weekend. I fix my favourite foods. Eat. Turn off the phone and light some scented candles or incense. I sink into a tub of hot bubbles and a good book. Sometimes when my burden is heavy and Billie Holiday hits that lonesome note, I cry. I wrap my arms around my own body in praise of your memory and myself.

A Better Woman Because of It

CJAJDIANN M. HARRIS

Bilateral salphingo oophorectomy. There, if I learned to say it (which of course I would); if I could make it roll off my tongue; if I could make it become an integral part of my conversation and thought, then perhaps I could accept and understand it.

When said altogether, you can disregard *bilateral*, focus on *salphingo*, which sounds almost romantic and tempers *oophorectomy* which is the ugliest word I've ever heard. If I had to have an operation, why not the laproscopy? It sounds much better. Why the big one? After all, I'm not the kind of person who has *knife* surgeries! "Please, God, don't let me be one of those women who have fifty different operations to compare and bore with. Don't let this be the beginning of the dreaded female-trouble-syndrome." Despite the fact that I can be associated with such words as: cystoscopy, orthroscopy, stillbirth, and rheumatoid arthritis (since age 24); "please, God, not the slice-'n-dice procedures, not me. I picked too good from the gene pool for this to be happening."

I've never had a bit of trouble with my periods. As a matter of fact, back in the day I even changed my cycle using the pill so that I never had my period during the weekend. I started on Monday and by Friday evening, I was clear to fly. So, now, wasn't I in charge of this business, here?

I had known that I had this thing growing inside of me for the last five years and it hadn't killed me yet. (For this I gave thanks to God and blame to jobs with no medical coverage, and a country with no national health care policy). Because I could do nothing about it, I purposed in my heart that I didn't *need* to do anything about it.

So, part of my defence mechanism was denial that misinformed and endangered me and had me thinking that I would never join that league of women – that group of poor unfortunates who were no longer whole unto themselves.

I managed to beat the oppressive system by taking a sales associate position in a women's clothing store, specifically because they were owned by a large corporation and offered medical as part of their benefit package. I waited patiently through my probationary period, and did not return to the cold, impersonal, ready-to-cut gynecologist who first cited the *alien* the size of an orange that had attached itself to my right ovary. I also did not want any paper trail and by going to a different doctor there was no chance that my new insurance could refuse to pay because this was a pre-existing illness. The new doctor that I so carefully selected to change my life was wonderful. She was my sex, my age, and my colour. She could have *been* me. How patiently she explained every detail and firmly, almost lovingly, she refused to take the other tube and ovary and just "get it over with", as I requested. She insisted that I still had time and might change my mind and decide to become pregnant. She also stressed the importance of allowing my body to continue the natural, healthy course of maturation and not be forced to take synthetic hormone replacement or throw my clock off by going into early menopause.

I felt secure in her care right up until the time I was rolled to the door of OR #3 and I burst into tears. She soothed me, rubbing my hand and asking if anyone had come with me. "No," I sobbed, trying to hypnotize myself by watching her wedding rings swing on the safety pin attached to her gown. "My sister went on to work because they told us you'd be awhile." She marched off to make sure my sister would be called immediately.

Dr. Wonderful had told me about pain from the incision and what kind of pain medication she would be prescribing. I couldn't conceive of being off work for six weeks, although she insisted. Despite all of her preparation, I still was not prepared. Neither my mind nor my heart was ready for the intrusion of surgical steel into my womanhood, and the truth is, I could never be prepared. However, someone should have told me that I would want to die from all of the air in my abdomen afterwards. Not only was there excruciating physical pain; there was also mental anguish, the harsh reality that I had been opened, actually laid open and exposed. Had part of my soul escaped? Who would I be now that part of me was gone?

A year and a half later, I'm still me. I'm me – only better. Older, wiser, more focused and determined than I've ever been. No, I don't attribute it to an operation, but it is the direct result of, once again, having to do something I absolutely did not want to do. Having to do what was best for me, having to be my own parent, caring for myself, and I'm a better woman because of it.

Reprinted with permission by CiajDiann Harris from her anthology entitled: *I Count it All Joy*. Copyright 2000.

Endo Poems

ROSAMOND S. KING

first the fever

the whole air is baking you
water makes steam with your skin
then the mud snakes
and the pain starts (behind the intestines
in the back) it all keeps you
sitting in a small room
forehead against the cool wall
all this before blood
which will come in two days time
groping for ibuprofen
through it all your mouth is closed
even when the pain is a small animal
chewing an oval perimeter in your flesh
because those whose ears can hear
the telling of this woman's thing
will make their eyes small
to see if you are creating demons
for yourself or maybe just writing poems
throughout it all your mouth is closed
even if it sinks you to the ground deflated
even then no sounds are made
because the truth is on the inside of your flesh
and the best that those who believe can say is
"there is no cure"

Endo 4
The punctuation in between
the fact that you manage to function
is twisted from necessity to proof
of deception and wasting everyone's time
as if buildings all in white are amusement
parks; strangers' hands on your body are the ferris wheel
cold hard silver between your legs cotton candy

What do you do with a body abused by medicine?
 The greater wrong is not the side
  effect but that you do not know who
   you would have been.
    Suck out all the fat. Cut off
     your hair. Wear a wig. Ask
      those who could not heal you
       to help you again and
        you will not be who
         you would have been.
          just someone else
           again.

4am Descent

my mind is skiing
    fast
    fast
don't want to fall down down
waver
    between I am falling
    and I am fiiiine
no one will make the metaphor
    ever say she is like finery
    thin and easily broken
this woman be big
this woman be strong
she ain't no flower
do you take tablets to sleep?
I won't have
    pills and alcohol in my
    house says the chichidodobird
it is only your stench
that keeps me awake
    chichidodobird
        the stench is you

out me under
a knife then
if I'm all
wrong
put me to sleep
with gas but
I won't have
pills and alcohol
in my house

they ask you to write
    a journal
    to "keep" one
    when they don't believe
        your pain

    I know
blood on the page
is not enough
    in some time
        though
    I'll smear it
around make
you think I've got
an ochre pen

The corps is whole • unto itself with • all its holes and gashes • there
is no meaning beyond *this* flesh • it is whole cut • open and sewn up •
scarred weakened • pieces missing • in chronic pain • *this* body is as •
whole as that one • *this* body is • not wrong dis un • *this* • *whole* • body
holds a • full person brilliant • to bursting

Help, I've Fallen, and No One Has Even Noticed

JUDITH K. WITHEROW

When I was diagnosed with multiple sclerosis in 1979, my neurologist told me to avoid stress. I didn't take his advice seriously. Stress was one of those middle-class words that lost something in translation to real life. Throughout my story you will see an over abundance of stress. At this late date, it occurs to me that avoiding stress wasn't my mission. Understanding, managing, and confronting it in ways that related to my lifestyle were the answers I needed.

Years ago, when I was working on an article, I discussed our family history with my mother. I needed her input to uncloud my memory about many of our childhood ailments and customs. I specifically wanted to know about many of the superstitions.

She informed me she didn't know of any superstitions. I asked, "What about when you were a baby and whooping cough was going around? You told us your parents took you to a neighbour who had a black stallion and had it blow its breath in your face. Because of that belief, you were protected." "That wasn't a superstition," she replied. "It worked."

Another treatment that worked: when one of us would step on a nail and injure our foot, Mother would always grease the nail and put it over the front door. She said, "If any evil spirits come in they will slide back out and you won't get an infection."

Her kind looks turned to a blank stare as I continued asking questions. It was the type of look you'd give a census taker or social worker. Someone, who knew nothing about you, but insisted on cramming you into a one-size-fits-all mould. I became the dreaded stranger who brought fear and embarrassment in through the front door. By saying out loud what our life had been like, and calling it superstitious, I brought shame to her.

If I had been as kind and wise as she always was, I would have phrased my questions differently. (She died on November 24, 1992). Better yet – I wouldn't have discounted our culture so cruelly. We have a saying that every pig has to burn its own snout. Without a doubt I will forever bear the scars of that experience.

The environment wasn't an easy subject to discuss either. Since we didn't live in a house that had running water until after I was fourteen years old, I wanted to talk about our own water supply. Mom said our drinking water couldn't have been polluted because it always looked clean. The only *polluted* water Mom remembered hearing about was a dead rat that was found in the town reservoir. Many things in our life were, and always will be, a simple matter of faith.

Our water came out of a wooden trough, embedded in a hillside, which had been strip-mined for coal years earlier. The abandoned mine shaft near it was one of our favourite places to play. Runoff from the mines around our small town turned the river reddish yellow and killed the fish and other living things. Who knew what poisons these mines exuded or what they would do to humans? (Years later the mine owners were forced by law to plant trees and treat the water.) Human loss, and disease, was another matter. I hear frequent stories of cancer and multiple sclerosis and other immune system disorders. Their cause is rarely discussed or believed.

This was the background we emerged from. Myths, superstitions, lack of education, and poverty coated us like a cocoon and protected us from nothing.

There were eighteen children in my father's family. Some died at birth, others made it until childhood. Thirteen lived to be adults. Dad was born in rural Georgia and was of Cherokee blood. He quit school in the third grade to help support his family. He remains the smartest man I have ever known.

Mother was one of eleven children and one miscarriage. Her family lived in the Appalachian Mountains of Pennsylvania. She was

Seminole and Irish. Mom finished the seventh grade and grieved forever over her lost education.

We were raised in the area of my mother's birth. There were six live births and one miscarriage. I have three sisters and two brothers.

My earliest memories are of us living in a little three-room shack that had no electricity or water. Mom washed our clothes out back in the creek. The creek was also our "*refrigerator*" Racoons and other animals would often steal the food stored there. The food would also spoil or become saturated with water. Although Mom canned food and other family members fished and hunted, there never was enough food to eat. Hunger was a way of life I never became used to.

Winters were brutal. There were never enough clothes or bed-covers to generate warmth. Snow blew in through the cracks in the walls as well as around the windows and under the doors. Anything that would burn was placed in the wood stove; this included car tires. The smell was horrendous, and the stove would turn bright red from the heat. It's a miracle that the house didn't catch fire.

At the age of two, I was diagnosed as having a tapeworm. It's a worm made up of many segments and the sections keep breaking off. The head attaches itself to the stomach and grows to many feet in length. It was thought that I got mine from eating raw meat. When you are constantly hungry everything can be a temptation.

Needless to say, my parents tried many home remedies. Anything suggested as a cure was given to me. I recall drinking quarts of sauerkraut juice. Another supposed cure was coconut milk. Since these items weren't part of our diet I can only assume they were thought of as exotic enough to work. They didn't.

Doctors suggested mixing kerosene or turpentine with sugar on a tablespoon, and having me eat it. They told Mom if the tapeworm got hungry it would come up in my throat and choke me. With hindsight, I see that her cures were safer than those of the medical establishments.

At age ten I was hospitalized with scarlet fever. I remember being acutely ill for two weeks. During the third week, doctors adminis-tered an experimental medicine to cure me of my tapeworm. My parents were told that if they would give their permission, no bill would be owed for my stay. Since these doctors were *educated*, they had to know what was best. The medicine was so harsh that a rubber tube was inserted in my nose and pushed down into my stomach. Even so, when the medicine was given, I started to vomit. I don't know what the medicine was, but it did kill the tapeworm.

When generation after generation is caught in a web of poverty, alcoholism, numerous health problems, and very little formal education, it becomes almost impossible to take control of your life. While there might be small pockets of change, the vast majority does not escape.

My parents worked extremely hard all of their lives. Dad was a carpenter. Mom cleaned other people's houses and did factory work. After graduation from high school in 1962, I joined my older sister and mother at the same textile factory.

The factory was hot in the summer and cold in the winter. Cotton dust was so thick that you could barely catch your breath, and the noise from the sewing machines was deafening. I developed several allergies while working there. I was seventeen years old at that time. Several women had complete breakdowns while working. When we would hear the screaming we would sew faster as if to outrun the demons. No one ever raised their head from their work. You didn't want to know if it was one of your kin.

With a number of us working and helping out at home, our quality of life improved. We were able to buy a cheap house in town. It had electricity and running water. We lived there for about five years. In 1964 the house caught fire. A faulty pump that pumped the water up from the well caused it. The fire didn't do much damage but the firefighters did. They used their hatchets to destroy just about everything we had. What couldn't be chopped up was soaked with water. Since Dad was a carpenter, we decided to repair the house. We took all of the trash to the dump and we were going to start rebuilding the next day. That night someone poured gasoline throughout the house and burned it to the ground. There were witnesses, but no one wanted to become involved. They said, "they had to live there." I guess the way they looked at it we could live anywhere.

Our move to Maryland, in 1964, was one of the best family decisions we ever made. It exposed us to city life and showed a range of class, race, and culture that we didn't know existed. You could blend in or stand out at will. Our customs of hunting, fishing, and food gathering could still be practiced here.

I married before leaving Pennsylvania. In our family, you married, had children, and lived your life within the family. You didn't view yourself as an individual. The man I married was a white man.

As we grow older our health problems increase. First Nation people have the worst health statistics of any race. Be it alcoholism, drug abuse, poverty, suicide, disease, you name it, if it's a hardship, it will be inherited. Among my mother, father, sisters, and brothers, we all have some form of arthritis. The men have alcohol problems. Most of us have asthma, emphysema, or chronic bronchitis. All have some form of skin disease, including melanoma, vitiligo, psoriasis, or eczema. Diabetes, heart disease, gall bladder disease (two-thirds of First Nation people have gall bladder disease), endometriosis, high blood pressure, ulcers, Parkinson's, and atherosclerosis affect most of the family. Cancer of all types is now occurring. (My father died of lung cancer in 1990). I have multiple sclerosis and systemic lupus erythematosus. One of my brothers shows signs of developing multiple sclerosis.

All three of my sons have learning disabilities, as do most of our children and grandchildren. My oldest son has cardio-pulmonary sarcoidosis, diabetes, and high blood pressure. The middle son had hepatitis. (He caught it from fishing in polluted waters.) He has also had mononucleosis, and continues to have numerous infections. My neurologist says the likelihood of his developing MS is great. The youngest son has always had severe hay fever, food and bee sting allergies, and vitiligo.

I am appalled as I write this. I thought this generation would be able to overcome past obstacles because the quality of our life has improved considerably. A full plate can feed the body, but it doesn't necessarily follow that it will repair the past deficiencies of malnutrition. Jesus! What we assumed was continuing bad luck is even more sinister.

During the ten years that I was married I gave birth to three children. With each pregnancy there was a noticeable decline in my health. Often, my legs would weaken and I would stumble and fall. Doctors diagnosed my symptoms with every lame guess they could think up.

In 1972, I gave birth for the last time. It was a difficult pregnancy. I had a seizure in the eighth month. My obstetrician didn't want his patients to gain more than twenty pounds so he put me on Dexedrine, a diet pill. There were many days that I couldn't even force myself to eat a cookie. When I had the seizure, another doctor took over my care.

Neurological symptoms kept occurring, but they would disappear before I could get an appointment with a doctor.

In 1974, after months of gastrointestinal ailments, my gall bladder was removed. There was a very slow recovery. Throughout all of this, I was having frequent, painful, hemorrhaging periods.

In 1975, I was told I had endometriosis. Premarin was tried, but it didn't help. Then I had a D & C. The pain and hemorrhaging continued. I had a hysterectomy. It seemed radical, but it stopped the bleeding. Unfortunately, it didn't stop the growths on my ovaries.

The hysterectomy escalated the violence in my marriage. I apparently needed my uterus to prove that I was a real woman.

In the summer of 1976, I met Sue, my partner for the past twenty-four years. With Sue's help I took the three boys and moved into an apartment in the District of Columbia. The house I left was sold, and I received half of the money and custody of the three boys.

During March 1977, I was having severe pain in my side. Tests showed a large tumour where my left ovary should have been. The endometriosis was back. Surgery was done to remove the tumour and part of my right ovary where another growth had started.

In October of 1977, the pain in my right ovary became so painful that I was hospitalized. The surgeon wanted to save part of the ovary, but I insisted that all of it be removed. This piecemeal surgery was destroying me mentally and physically. I also refused estrogen therapy. There were dire warnings about being "thrown into the change of life" overnight. It occurred, but I managed it with vitamins. Sue and I researched what vitamins would relieve the hot flashes, night sweats, and mood swings. The regimen worked.

During the surgery, I later found out, the doctor had sutured my right ureter closed. When I kept complaining of the pain, and that something was very wrong, the doctor released me and refused to see me again. The next time he saw me was when I sued him and won.

Two months later in December of 1977, I had major reconstructive surgery to remove four inches of my right ureter. It was then reimplanted in the bladder. A valve to prevent reflux into the kidney was also fashioned. It worked for a short while. Because the kidney was closed off for so long, a large nephrosis had occurred. I was told that two-thirds of my kidney wasn't functioning, and the left kidney was swollen because of the overload. After each surgery I would have bouts of pins and needles in my hands, stumbling, numbness, and many other symptoms diagnosed as anemia or stress.

I had ongoing urinary problems that continued into 1978. That April, because of blood in my urine, I was hospitalized again. While there, I asked the doctor to look at a mole on my foot that looked suspicious.

A biopsy found that it was a malignant melanoma, and a section of my foot was removed. With this type of cancer you can have just one or five hundred. You can also pass the tendency to develop melanoma on to your children.

The numbness and pins and needles were more frequent now. It was decided that I should be given two transfusions of platelets, that I was anemic.

A new symptom developed: a burning pain in my spine. X-rays were negative. My urologist was a great guy. He kept saying, "Judith, I know you are having all of these symptoms, but I swear it's not a urinary problem."

One afternoon in April of 1979, I was overwhelmingly tired so I took a nap. During the sleep, I dreamed a wild bird was in the house. We were trying to get it outside without hurting it. (A wild bird in the house is a very bad omen). I woke up terrified.

When I tried to stand up, I discovered my left side was paralysed from my eye down to my foot. Sue took me to the emergency room. They gave me the name of a neurologist to call for an appointment.

On my first appointment, a basic neurological exam was conducted. The doctor tested my sense of touch, smell and hearing. I followed an object's movement with my eyes and walked a straight line to see if gait variations were evident. Many things were tried to elicit the correct response from the brain.

I then had an EEG. While I was trying to get the paste out of my long hair, the doctor went out to speak with Sue in private. He told her he thought the melanoma had spread to my brain and the chances of survival were slim. She was also told not to tell me.

Naturally, she told me right away. We were devastated. Every other time there had been hope, but this time called for the planning of an ending not a recovery. I made out a will and a medical power of attorney that gave Sue medical decision-making powers.

When a CAT scan of the brain showed no evidence of a tumour, the diagnosis was changed to a stroke.

A month later I had another episode of paralysis. My vision and speech were also effected. A physical therapist made me promise I wouldn't let anyone try to tell me it was my imagination. She knew that women were often suspected of having an over active imagination – particularly women of colour.

I made a decision to change doctors. I was hospitalized, and the testing began again. A lumbar puncture was done. It was the sickest week of my life. I couldn't get out of bed. Every time I sat up I started to vomit. It took a week for the needle stick to heal. This test and other observations gave a firm diagnosis. I had multiple sclerosis: the great crippler of young adults. (Diagnosis has now been made easier with MRI, magnetic resonance imaging).

In 1981, I had the worst MS exacerbation to date. I was in the hospital for five and a half weeks. No part of my body seemed exempt from damage. During this time, I developed many opportunistic infections that weakened me further. I was unable to walk, and spasticity developed in both arms and legs. They brought me home in a wheelchair, and it looked like I would remain in one. I required home nursing care. This was what I thought all people with MS could expect. I wish someone had told me that every case was different and that many people with MS never needed a wheelchair. It would have lessened the worry considerably.

Throughout this time, everyone kept telling me to reduce the stress in my life. Testimonials will verify that my idea of stress prevention is in itself stressful. I am not a quiet person. I am not a calm person. Isn't that what stress reduction means? Leaving my husband allowed me to find my voice and I want my words to echo forever.

During this ordeal, everyone, including doctors, would say, "you don't look sick, you look good." It has become a long-standing joke among us that whenever a new health crisis occurs, we say, "but you look good." A compliment instead of a cure doesn't seem like an equal trade, but hey, that's just my opinion.

It has been twenty-two years since I was diagnosed with multiple sclerosis. The doctor responsible for the diagnosis continued to treat me even though I was on SSI and medical assistance. When he became interested in research, he assumed that I would be a willing subject. Someone who once was a caring person turned into one of the most callous people I have ever known. In 1999 I found another neurologist. I view him with cautious eyes that cut deeper than a scalpel.

One of the most aggravating health problems I have is a skin disorder. For seven years it was diagnosed as just about everything. Several doctors mistakenly called it eczema, despite the characteristic discoid shape of lupus lesions. In fact, the *eczema* was one of the early signs of collagen vascular disease and SLE, yet another sign of my immune system's failure. I ordered, and paid for, an anti-nuclear antibody biopsy on one of the lesions. This led to the correct diagnosis. My general practitioner remarked, "you already had one incurable disease and I didn't want you to be diagnosed with another." In another life, if there is any justice, our roles will be reversed.

I thought, when I started this article, that I could contribute some insight into dealing with incurable illnesses. However, I have gained more than I have given. Putting everything down in black and white has given me the answers to questions I have been asking for years.

We all say, "I know just how you feel," when discussing someone's illness. No, you don't. You can empathize, and hopefully educate yourself, but that's as close as you'll get. I know that I have gained the bulk of my knowledge from experience. Sharing information with others who are battling MS and SLE has helped considerably. None of us have the same group of numerous changing symptoms. Reading everything I can find and staying up-to-date on research helps greatly. Don't believe that your doctor has the time to stay up-to-date on everything.

Guilt, anger, fear, and sadness are natural parts of any illness. You are entitled to these feelings. Between the incurable illnesses you have, and the medicines to control some of the symptoms, your moods can alter radically. Steroids are particularly their own living hell.

A good sense of humour can be a blessing. It can put others at ease when they are feeling helpless, and it can help you maintain your sanity when the unpredictable nature of any disease gets to be too much. Don't worry, "you look good!"

Learn that medical equipment can make life easier. It's not an admission of disability; it's just common sense. I use a cane (a flashy engraved green one), and I'll use whatever it takes to keep me as mobile as possible.

My greatest fear is for the future: not mine but that of my sons, grandchildren, and that of my families. Scientists now know that there are familial links to many diseases. Knowing ahead of time that you could acquire a particular disease might not alter the course of it, but it could ease the nightmare of trying to get a firm diagnosis sooner.

I need to believe that with all of the research being done on AIDS, a cure for other immune system disorders, including MS, Parkinson's, and SLE will be found.

There is now the overwhelming realization of what my family is facing. Not a quick, certain death but a slow torturous one that will be endured for time without end.

I cannot repair the ongoing damage to the earth. Nor will I try to replace family superstition with the harsh words of truth. I will watch and wait like those in the government. But unlike the government, I will assist and ease the suffering whenever possible. When the time is right I will pass this knowledge on to another. I will whisper that it is not evil spirits or bad luck. It is much, much scarier than that.

During the writing of this article tests showed that my right kidney has stopped functioning. My health is too compromised to have it removed. The powers that be will make a decision, and I will try to see what options are available. My list of daily medicines increased to fourteen. Some of them need to be taken two or three times a day. I'm on my third type of chemotherapy. If I had it to do over, I would have never agreed to some of these treatments or medicines. They have caused their own set of symptoms and side effects. In particular, I would have stayed away from any form of chemo. The desire to live, and have some of the pain kept under control, reinforces my knowledge that I really didn't have an adequate choice.

The Sunday before I went to the urologist I had a dream about being in a hospital bed. I was holding the x-ray films of my kidney exam. Mom, I wish you were here to impart words of wisdom. I am so sorry that I ever used the word "superstition."

Secrets

NOAMI NORTH

I do not notice
the gradual changes
my body marks
holding on
to intangible despair

I wake up
charged by grief
and the heavy weight
my body sounds
as spine buckles
in resonance

It is easy to forget
i am woman
with secrets to joy
body holding heart
in hand transformed
by witness to terror

Vertigo of knowledge
keeping me breathless
and searching
for escape

So silently
tonight
i linger
and gently
raise my arms
relinquish
to an expansive night air.

Generations

NOAMI NORTH

We are woven
voices in this
tapestry
care given to
the intertwining
of complimentary
threads
illustrating detailed
histories and
dreams of
lives lived
and though
perhaps forgotten
imprinting
demands for justice
in my memory.

Fairy Tales and Bedtime Stories

LAYLA HASSAN

#1

I was a woman you know
At the age of nine,
But the Cancer was up my pelvis creeping, crawling
When I wasn't looking.

It was me: a child in woman's gear,
six months experiments, six months of fear.
Grown child in a dish
For examination of the drugs
To save my life without a kiss.

At age eleven I had no breasts
They shrunk away and left.
Grateful I accepted this
My one and only wish.

I sat in tears of reality as they slammed straight down my face
Take away my dirty pubic hair
Please don't leave a trace
But pushed away the suffocating
Bath of water snakes.

I prayed through the pain
Then swore at God and prayed again.
Just let me look like skinny Stephanie,
She's smooth as butter not a trace of dark
White as paper bark.

The second time they cut me up
Thoughts of murder from an eleven year old mind
Dreams dark and grim
Scared as the elephant man
Fists tight, I was never to win.

The game was up
My thigh gone, my ass a bloody mess
I am awake, yes.
Sleep now, the princess said.
Life awaits you, not death.

#2

Terry Fox, what good were you to me
"Amputee brother"?
You'll never catch me
Sweating for money I'll never see.

With corporate bucks around
Hospital still shuts down
And where will you be Sir,
When the shit goes down?

Breasts, liver, rectum, colon
Body parts abducted and stolen
Like Snickers from the candy store
A child from her mother's door.

Stomach, blood, lung and brain
Pain to drive a rock insane
Bones and bowels broke in half
By hands excelling at their craft.

The cancer of the rich
In her tanning stations
Meet the cancer of the poor
In the poorest nations

Global conspiracies
Patents on land
White hate strong
Power of quick sand.

They might bury you with sterility pills,
Birth control and Pamprin
While their dicks get hard on Viagra
Women are in season.

Incestuous governmental scientists
With sticky little fingers
Putting their paws where they don't belong
On the lands/blood of Native peoples.

Chemo for cancer kids
Organic food and clean air?
Not a lot of that to spare
Our fine ministers must have their share.

Hair loss, diarrhea, herpes and constipation
Punishment equal to damnation.
Nowhere to go, nothing inside
Hospital beds don't have places to hide.

I.V. in my arm till death do us part
Bags of barf in the corner
Where once sat alone
A boy called little Jack Horner

Transfusions and surgeries
MD's pathologies and corporate junkies
All hiding under the bed
Wait till she's asleep, they said.

And when everything was ready,
Like a thief in the night,
They stole my hair, and my smile,
But only for a while.

The end.

Bone Doctor

HEATHER MACLEOD

He leans over me,
wraps his arms around me,
tells me to drop my left shoulder
and my chin, take a deep breath
and then my spine is moved,
adjusted into its proper place.
He moves me like a rag doll,
swings my head from side to side,
crosses my arms over my chest,
lifts my leg, tells me to roll over,
leans against me, lifts my other leg,
the endless adjusting and aligning,
but it all sounds like cracking to me.
The evocative music of my bones;
the way he sees me as a series
of knotted calcium, a connection of sockets,
a braid of bone fitting, not fitting
and how he is called to me, every day
for him a celebration of the dead,
to lean over not flesh and tendon,
not my old bra with the lace stretched
against my nipples, to him I'm all skeleton;
a celebration of sun-bleached bone.
His hair is gnarled leaps of yellow,
his breath fresh and cold over my neck
and spine, against my cheek;

he murmurs as he moves over me,
his hands at my buttocks, adjusting
my out of place hips;
my long hair falls forward,
hangs down by my hands; him up
behind me, just a series of touches
and leanings, a series of murmurs;
my hair smells of sesame seeds.
I imagine his warm brown hands
against flesh and muscle,
but all he feels are my bones.

Token of Chastity

HEATHER MACLEOD

"... these are the tokens of my daughter's virginity."
Deuteronomy 22:17

Sometimes I dream, I gather a child from the water just as Moses was gathered from the water. Dreams move and push aside all other cognitive thoughts. My dream life is sometimes richer than this moving-awake existence, and dreams take what I know, what I've remembered, what I've forgotten and gather the knowledge of myself together like clothes-pegs in the mouth. I can barely speak words around all I used to know, all I've forgotten, and pieces of what I've remembered.

I want to hold life in my hands, but holding life is like holding water. Water searches out crevices and points of escape, and cannot be contained.

****

In the beginning I refused to remember, I pulled a woollen blanket over my mind and said, "This I cannot hold," and I searched out a crevice and I hid it.

And the little girl I was then, at that moment, sat still and watched guard against a memory that couldn't be held. She pushed it back inside the crevice with a long stick every time it tried, like water, to escape. So, in her absence, she was forced to create another in our own image to go forth in the light of day.

She named me, Heather.

My grandmother speaks to me. She asks, "When will you marry?" And I hear birds in the rafters (*If any man take a wife, and go in unto her, and hate her*) sailing in the air (*And give occasions of speech against her, and bring up an evil name upon her*) flying like fish swim in water (*and say, I took this woman, and when I came to her*) one clean stroke after another (*I found her not a maid*) with no regret.

My grandma sees me as an old crone. My red hair, to her eyes, is white and gray. Hair that cannot hold its youth, but shuns it. In her eyes I am shrunken; made small as regret. She says to me, "Why don't you have a fella?" And I hear waterfalls (Then shall the father … take and bring forth the tokens of the damsel's virginity). I need enough water to bury me, and silence all my grandmother's questions. Please (But if this thing be true, and the tokens of virginity be not found for the damsel) let water fall over me (Then they shall bring out the damsel) there (the men of her city shall stone her with stones that she die: because) be fresh as mountain air (she hath wrought folly … to play the whore in her father's house) and let there be enough.

*****

The heart of woman is deeper than the deepest sea in the world – Breton proverb from the Île de Batz

I want my father to bring me tokens of my virginity. I was made maiden long before I was ready, and so I have been woman when I should have been girl.

The sheet he bled me on must long be forgotten. Not even I can remember its fabric or pattern. Not even I remember the blood. But does he? If I go to him now, with rocks in my hands and the chill of my breath, will he know why I have come so far? Will he, like God, watch me walk along the hot sand (the quiver of my stride) and he, like God, watch with indifference? Or will he run about his house, gather the replacement family about him, wave his arm as I approach and barely whisper, "Shoo … shoo." Run his hand along the water that drips down his neck in the heat of another day, and think to himself: I barely remember her. Think to himself: All I know of her is her name.

And I will, as I always do, stop strides from his house. My heels blistering in the sand, blow my breath down my shirt to cool my skin and I think: Why have I come so far? I think: I do not know this one. He has nothing for me. It is then, while I'm still thinking – I have never even called him 'Father' – that I feel God. Feel my tongue running along God's mouth, feel my hands against his flesh and then I think: I have come so far – for nothing. I leave the rocks at his doorstep, and turn myself toward another day.

****

Because I love(d) him I couldn't sleep with him. Couldn't make my body let him have it. I wanted him to have me, but I d(idn't)on't know what that mean(t)s.

Instead I let him loose like water; followed him through the waves; dreamed I could be a mermaid to his fish. Filled myself endlessly with the dream.

Stop dreaming. Stop dreaming and pining away the days. I hear the Everly Brothers everywhere I go. Everywhere I go. The Everly Brothers are singing to me.

I don't want to sleep anymore. I want to throw stones at my father. I want to throw stones across the water, and feel myself skipping across the white arc of waves, and feel myself falling. Falling like one small stone.

The men I've fucked are different. I pulled them inside me without much thought. Still, only, half awake. Some of them have told me I sleep with my eyes open, and I'm always surprised (and disappointed) to find them in the morning. Part of me doesn't understand why they don't slip out in the middle of the night when I've had my fill of them. *What are they thinking?*

Small talk is the worst. I have so little to say. I tell them lies, but mix everything up with the truth. Sometimes it seems I'm the only one confused.

Sometimes I become *angry* that I had to see them in the morning, and had to look at their faces. I feel angry that I had to smile, and pretend (pretend, pretend, pretend) and, so, I steal things in the afternoons (on my coffee break). I go into bookstores and boutiques where the shop girls know me. I take things right in front of them. Even while we're talking, I'm stealing. Sometimes big books that barely fit in my bag. I don't even care. I take whatever I want and I leave with my heart pounding and my blood boiling and my mind drifting over clear ponds – smiling.

***

One morning I saw how I'd stained my bedding with my monthly blood. I saw as I pulled the bedding from the mattress that I'd stained even that. I cut the cloth of my blood out and flipped the mattress. Then I glued the blood-soaked fabric in my journal. I dreamed I brought the fabric to my father's new house, in the desert. I dreamed I walked a thousand miles in the burning heat and when I came to his house he didn't recognize me. Didn't even know who I was. So when I handed him my blood-soaked fabric he said, "What is this?" And in my dreams I tell him, "This is the token of your daughter's chastity."

**

If I could design and shape my own beginnings I would have my father find me in a river outside his house. He would bend with some surprise, but not too much, and look closely at me. I would look back, and my mother would raise her head from her garden and call out, "What do you see?" And my father would call back to her, "A lovely flower," and then he would turn his back upon me and walk toward my mother smiling. And I would drift down the Nile – sleeping with my eyes open.

When I die it'll be in the water. Christ will be swimming ahead of me, urging me to follow him. I will. I'll follow him down to the blackest part of the ocean, and when he stops and tells me, "I'm a man and can't go any farther. Only women's grief goes deeper." I'll keep swimming until I see her, the glint of her hunting knife tucked in the belt at her waist. I'll close my eyes, take a deep breath, and awaken.

Four Forces

VALERIE WOOD

Rain
washes the earth
as tears
cleanse the heart
of sorrow.

Moon
lights the circle
as fires
accept prayers
of thanksgiving.

Sun
warms the earth
as creation
sings her song
of celebration.

Earth
is the provider
as mother
suckles her child
of creation.

Windows

VALERIE WOOD

Through hazy panes of grief,
she stands alone.
The horizon clouds over,
she is swallowed.
Down her youthful brown face,
salty rivers trail.
In a baby-swollen belly,
grows tomorrow.
Her voice like her belly,
grows stronger.
Despair and resignation,
once her companion fade.
Windows open,
giving way to hope.
In that firm round belly,
lives promise.
Thrusting her chin skyward,
in defiance of her past.
She looks boldly to tomorrow,
wiping away happy tears.
Patting her full belly,
chatting to the baby.
At least for today,
her demons rest.

Freeing the Inner Child

VALERIE WOOD

A quiet internal rage
    rains skepticism
        on a private parade
            of fleeting childhood dreams.

A red hot sensation
    drives emotion
        into the forefront
            begging to be seen.

A flat resolve
    blocks those tears
        that await to release
            to travel down her cheeks.

A silent scream
    struggles against
        the crumbling wall
            needing to be heard.

A heavy sorrow
    like fingerling fog
        swirls its way
            around a wounded heart.

A weary soul
        searches the keys
                to free the inner child
                        that only she holds.

Wolf Cry

LORRAINE THOMAS

May your heart be
All that I dreamed of
Loyal and wild
Like that of a wolf
Who hunts in the night
Who howls his lonely wolf cry
At the same blue moon
In faith I wait
In this empty den
For it is I
Your mate
In the moonlit lands

Erect in Green Pride

LORRAINE THOMAS

In the army
Is a green rainbow
Warriors supposedly ungendered
Like wise boys and wo/men

But two hands extended
The Native and non
On each finger
They counted the reasons

What will you do
When there is another Oka
Indians fighting Indians
For the sake of the queen

What will you do
If I am a racist
If I don't accept you
Especially brown female skin in green

I wanted to scream for humanity
Go to war against racism
Stand firm in combat boots
Stand erect in green pride

Anjali

BISHAKHA CHOWDHURY

As autumn sunlight
faded to dark night
a beautiful child
was born
Not ready
for this world yet
she died

My womb
which, every month
from thirteen years,
sheds tears of blood
for destiny unfulfilled
Now mourns desolately
spilling tears of blood
in a sorrow
only she can know

And the love
which held my daughter
safely
Becomes, slowly,
the love
which lets her go
the love
which gives Anjali
—offering—
to the
great, wide cosmic

Untitled

BISHAKHA CHOWDHURY

in the winter deep
new buds on the hawthorne tree
promise of new life

The Struggle of One and Many

ROXANE TRACEY

In dedication of Shadane Arone.
Rest in peace.

One day I realized I never knew your name
so I wondered about your dreams
caged by the colonial fists
which had sealed your eyes shut
pushing their hatred
into the warm dark spaces
of the back of your mind
One day I realized I never knew your story
Because the newspapers never spoke
of the burden on your back
the one underneath your skin
which bore the bruises of your exploitation
But instead made you a photo of black bruises
bruised blackness
which becomes most famous when it is
beaten
and especially when it
dies

Sad Paper

ROXANE TRACEY

Looking at this kleenex
it tells a story.

Its tiny fibers holding
the cool dampness
that my heart squeezed
out of the corners
of my eyes,
to plunk down
and out
like lonely piano chords
in the dark
it plays a
once-upon-a-time melody,
each tatter and wrinkle singing
a soft blues song
of sweet molasses love
that one day ran bitter
on the curve of my tongue.

It whispers a sorrow tale
told by
thousands of tiny
wishing-well pores
which can never seem
to hold enough tears.

My Aunt Patsy

TROY HUNTER

December 1999

My name is Troy Hunter and I am a member of the Ktunaxa Nation in southeast B.C. My stepdad was Willie Benallie. Willie was a champion boxer because he won a bronze medal in the Canada Winter Games in the mid-1970s. I have two brothers and I am the *middle-aged* son. My younger brother is Willie's true son. My stepdad Willie died in 1977 due to a drinking and driving accident. However, this story is not about Willie or my brothers, but about my Aunt Patsy who was Willie's older sister.

It must have been the spring of 1978 when Patsy moved in with us kids, along with her two oldest children Nina and Earl. My mom was still in the hospital recovering from her coma of the 1977 car accident. When Willie was alive, he was mean and abusive and we quickly learned that Patsy was not much different. Violence, drugs, and alcohol around the home was normal for us, and we inherited it from the previous generations.

Willie told us how his dad would tell him to get a thorny, wild rose branch, that was used when he needed to be disciplined; he took it easy on us kids as only a belt or crib board was used. Fear should never be part of a child's life, but our indigenous families have been broken by residential schools, the welfare system, and a myriad of abuses, to which I attribute drugs, alcohol, sexual abuse, and jealousy as major problems. There are deep levels of pain, abuse, and suffering. Memories stir the emotions and can bring back the hurt; some things are better left unsaid but some stories need to be shared.

Patsy's story was told to me in her small room overlooking one of Canada's poorest communities: Vancouver's Downtown Eastside. I

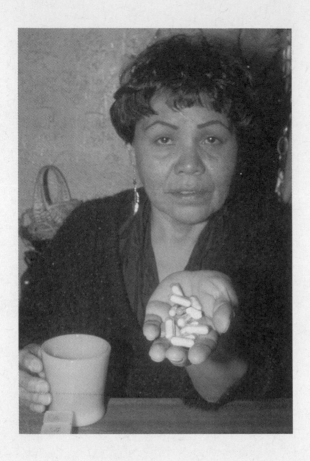

was walking along Hastings Street when I saw my Aunt Patsy walking towards me. We hadn't seen each other in almost twenty years,
but I immediately recognized her. I spoke Ktunaxa as we made eye
contact, as she tried to figure out who I was. It was rumoured that
Patsy had AIDS. When she finally realized who I was, I gave her a
big warm hug. Our chance encounter was probably destiny, as she
was hoping to find someone that would listen to her story. For Patsy,
telling her story is part of the healing journey that she is going
through. This is Patsy's story and she wants it to be told.

It must have been on my mind to locate Patsy. I had wanted to
photograph her because I knew she had AIDS and there was a photo
contest calling for pictures of women with AIDS. After much dis-

cussion with her and her family, Patsy agreed to participate. Her youngest daughters, Venus and Amethyst, as well as her common-law husband Ray, were also willing candidates. What began as a project to enter a photography contest ended up being part of a heal-ing journey for the family that I hold close to my heart, for they are also my family.

PATSY'S FAMILY BACKGROUND

Patsy Benallie was born in September of 1952 on the Lower Kootenay Indian Reserve at Creston, B.C. Her mother was Monica (Monique) Francis born of Nick Francis and Alice Jacobs (who came from Montana). Patsy's father was a full-blooded Navajo from Colorado, whose name was Paul James Benallie, and he would have been sixty when he passed away in 1984. Paul's father was Lee Benallie. Patsy's sister Irene was born in 1950 when her mother Monique was only sixteen years old. Willie was born in May of 1951. Sarah Francis is a daughter of Monique, whose father was Louie Basil, and is Patsy's youngest sister who was born in 1953. Phillip was a baby when he died of pneumonia, but Patsy heard that Thomas White (Patsy's step-dad) sat on him because he wasn't his kid. Monique married Thomas White. Thomas fathered Michael who was born January 1963 and David born December 1963; the two siblings were both born in the same year.

PATSY'S STORY IN HER OWN WORDS

My grandmother (Alyssa Francis) raised us for a few years. We called her mom. We stayed with our grandparents until we had TV, which was when I was four. Then, I was sent to the Vancouver General Hospital to get cured of Tuberculosis. I went there because I was a non-status Indian, yet my sister Sarah went to the Coqualeetza hospital because she was a status Indian. Coqualeetza was only for those with status. I stayed in Vancouver at the hospital with the white kids when I was only four years old until the time I was in grade two.

My memories from the hospital aren't much, just that it was clean, sterile, three meals a day, pills, pills, and more pills. There was nothing there, nothing to be happy about and nothing to be afraid of. I was lonely at first and probably cried a lot. My Uncle Frenchy came to visit me once while I was in there. I remember him bringing me comic books; Little Lulu and Tubby, those kinds of comics. I came to, and he just stood there for a while. I remembered who he was. We didn't show affection or happiness when we were kids so we didn't do that when I met him again. There was just nothing there; he gave me the comics and then he left.

Pretty much the only person that I had playtime fun with was the janitor. He was a bald headed guy in a white suit and always seemed to have a mop. I was isolated, I didn't like it, and there was nothing, there was nobody. It must have been four to six months that I spent in isolation. Finally, when I was healthy enough I was able to start school with the other kids. I was put in a dormitory with them.

A year before I was released, Irene my older sister came in. She couldn't understand a word of English and I had lost the Ktunaxa language. I had been in there two or three years already by then. So, when they came in they just threw us together in the same room. It wasn't fun at all and I was scared; I was in this room with this wild girl that couldn't understand English.

When we both got better, Irene and I were shipped back home to Creston. It was around Halloween 1960. I was eight years old when I was let out. We stayed in Creston with Monique (who was supposed to be our mother). That was when welfare was just beginning to be put into place. Us Benallies were the only ones on welfare, so we were the lowest ones on the status line. I remember people from the reserve were jealous of us because Monique would get welfare money. The women would get jealous of her because the guys would hang around as she had the money to buy the booze. Thomas would buy all kinds of booze and hide it under his mattress and what not.

I failed grade two when I stayed with Thomas and my mother. Later, I failed grade five and that was when welfare finally took us away. It was about 1965 when they sent us to the St. Eugene Indian Residential School near Cranbrook. Before we could get into the residential school, we had to stay at foster homes because non-status

Indians weren't allowed in there yet. They didn't know where to put us because there were no foster kids in town at that time; there were no Indian kids in town period, unless they were adopted.

When they started phasing out the residential school in the late sixties, all of us kids that came from families on welfare – status or not – started to get foster parents in town. We were the guinea pigs more or less. We were breaking trail for the kids that would be scooped up for adoption in town. We had to start going to school in town because they were starting to close the residential school. They built the St. Mary's school in Cranbrook in 1966, sixty-seven, and that was when everybody started getting bussed into town to go to school. That was when I joined the bugle band. It was also my first year in high school as I was in grade eight.

I used to travel with the bugle band. It was just to get away from the residential school, to have an outing and to travel. When I think about it, that is when I would have quit school, in grade eight or nine, but because I was non-status, I stayed in school. I had nowhere else to go. I graduated in 1971 at Mount Baker Senior Secondary School, also in Cranbrook. Out of thirty of us that started in grade nine, I was the only one that graduated.

After I finished with school, I went to work because I couldn't pay for my own medical and dental. That first year I got a job at the residential school on a youth project. There were thirteen of us working there. I worked the summer for Canada Manpower in seventy-two, and then went to secretarial school in Kelowna. That was the year ... it was a date rape and I didn't know what that was. I came to the city to give up my son for adoption. Back then the churches looked down upon unmarried women so I had to come to the city.

When I came here to Vancouver, I found a job right away. I worked for the Bank of Commerce in 1973, which is the year Jeremy was born. He was born in July. I worked through the following year when I met Nina's dad. I quit work to look after his kids. I had just given up my kid and I took in two of somebody else's that weren't mine. Raised them and then, after a few years, I had Nina and I worked. I always worked.

It wasn't until I got married that I decided that I wanted – had always wanted – to go to university; but I didn't just want to get married to anybody just so that I could have status, I didn't believe in that. I wanted to marry the person because I loved him, not for money or just for status. I got married in Frog Lake Reserve in Alberta in 1980 to my two youngest daughters' father.

I divorced in eighty-two; it was a wicked divorce battle. That is when I started going to university, after I divorced. I have always gone to school and worked at the same time until eighty-four when some bad stuff happened. I ended up getting gang-banged there and I just went back to drinking because of it. I said I would take one year off from university. I had twenty-two credits in a year and a half. I just needed eighteen more to get my university degree and I thought I would just take that one year off. I was going to try to get my head together and go to counselling, but it was a lot harder than that. It wasn't just the rape that I had to look at – my husband, boyfriends that I have had – I realized that it just wasn't those guys; I had to look back at family and that's when it got way too heavy. I realized that the incest and bad stuff that happened to us when growing up took a toll. The year that I thought I was going to take to get help was way too much, and I never went back to school. Now I kick myself and wish I just stayed that extra year, I would have got my eighteen credits.

I was studying English, Native American studies, physical education, and holistics. When I started university in eighty-two in St. Paul, Alberta, I had gone through two semesters and that is where I got chosen to go to San Diego for this holistic youth development conference. With the Elders wanting holistics involved, I was chosen to go and that is when I got involved with Phil Lane from the Four Worlds Project. That was the same time the Alkali Lake story got started, where they achieved 100 per cent sobriety in their community. At the same time, I didn't want to feel like a hypocrite; I didn't want to be teaching things when I wasn't practicing them myself. I couldn't talk about non-smoking, non-drinking, and non-drugging when I wasn't straight enough myself to not use it. I felt I shouldn't be in that position when I wasn't practicing what I preached.

My two youngest daughters are ragged, they are on the edge. It is as if they are waiting for the bomb to drop, it's like the death sentence sort of thing; although they know it's not that anymore. I think it's just them waiting for whatever, the unknown. I think its hard and they are trying to kill the pain as well, so they've gone to what I've been doing: heroin. They thought they could dabble in it. It's something you can't just dabble in, and it's taking its toll on their life, on our life.

The first year the doctors told me I was sick was in ninety-six. They said I wasn't going to live to see that Christmas. It took me ten days to try my suicide trip. On that one, I ended up getting four fractures and wound-up in the hospital. Oh, I wanted to die, I wanted to die.

I left the hospital after three days. I couldn't go in the bedpan. They threw that bedpan at me and told me to use it, but I kept getting up to go to the washroom; I couldn't do it in the bedpan. When they threw that at me and it hit me in the stomach is when I just got up and walked out. It took me an hour to walk from the top floor out to about a block away.

There was this little woman, a little white blond-haired woman, who had come along and saw me. She said, "Are you hurt, where are you going?" We were a block east down by the Army and Navy. She said again, "Are you hurt?"

I said, "yeah …" So she called a cab and gave the cabbie twenty bucks and said, "Give her a ride home and keep the change." It was a seven-dollar fare.

I went to the doctor the next day and got a bunch of T3s and Valium. That's what I did the first three months. I would just get up and go to the bathroom. That was probably the best thing for me. I should have been out of bed and just starting to walk at six months, but I was walking without my crutches at four months.

On July 1, 1996, I went on the Marijuana March. That was the first day I went without my crutches. I walked the complete march and it was hard. Indian women are tough. Indian women are really strong. We don't complain. We take a lot more pain than anyone I ever know and they hold it well. White women will take a lot longer to recover. It is good that I kept getting out of bed to go to the washroom and to get a drink of water, because that's the way we heal a lot faster.

I made my funeral arrangements. I waited but that time never came; I was getting sicker and sicker. After two years, I started taking the medication but it was too much. That was just before they started giving beepers out to the clients who are taking pills now. They never used to when I started, and it just gave me more harm than good. I was sick and frustrated and I just quit. I just didn't do any drugs. I don't know why I did it like that … oh, maybe it was because Elmer left. He went back to work up north and I had just met Ray.

I wasn't screwing around or running around like I used to. Elmer wouldn't wear a condom and I wouldn't let him without a condom, so we had a deadlock there. Finally he told me, just go find somebody and we could have lots, but without sex. I said, "okay" and that's how I met Ray.

In a way, I sort of felt obligated to stay with Ray. We used condoms for the first three weeks and then we didn't have any for a while there. He just didn't want to use them anymore. I told him that you are going to get sick, but he didn't care. Six months later, he came out positive. I wasn't really sure if I wanted to stay with him forever and ever, because I wasn't really sure if I had a future. I felt like I was obligated to stay with him because I passed the virus onto him. He says I can leave whenever, but now I don't want to be anywhere else. I feel good with him; I want to be with him.

It's hard to try to start a *family life* when you've never had it. I'm always looking for something; it's like when they say somebody threw a wrench in your motor. I always feel like something is going to go wrong. When it goes too good for long, I sort of … I have to wreck it. It's not quiet; it's supposed to be messed up according to my little mind. I'm not used to being bussed, or whatever. So, that's another big thing that the residential school did.

I got a hold of Charlie Chapin a couple of weeks ago. Ray and I had gone to an A.A. meeting with him but Ray's got a little thing with him. When I told him that I was going to use Charlie like my counsellor, or as my base to start my ship with the residential school project, he didn't think that was a good idea. I know I shouldn't be going by what he's feeling; I should be doing it for myself. That's where I feel like I'm still people crazy; I should be working on my own residential school project regards of how he feels, because he's never been through it. But, yet, I think I am using him as an excuse so I don't have to look at it. Once you start digging into that hole of the residential school, there is a lot of stuff that comes up. Unless you have a real good person that can take you out of a real deep feeling, hole, or whatever, you can be in a suicidal state for a while, so I have a hard time trying to get into that. You have to have a good safety net if you're going to get into that. I still have a lot of work to do and I'd like to get that started anyway.

One thing that Ray and I are looking forward to is Ray's land on an island, and what we are going to transform it into. We are going to be selling the timber off the island. We are going to look into the timber rights and start in the fall. We've got land, well timber coming in on that anyway. That is the other part of me there too; he wants to offer me whatever he has and I say "no, it's yours." It's my stubborn self, whether it makes sense or not, I am just stubborn or the wrong way. I know it can be worked out so that I don't wreck it. Maybe it can be a place for families that are sick, so they can get away for a month or a summer. They could do stuff like canning or fishing. I have got to get out of myself and start serving others. I get too much onto myself and I get onto pity.

I have some grandchildren now. I think it was March 1993 when I first became a grandmother. My grandkids and my oldest daughter came and visited me here in Vancouver in 1998. After they left is when I started using again. I just felt useless. I never saw them anymore after that. All I know is that my daughter is going to school and working in a bank out east somewhere, that's the last I heard anyway.

I worry about my kids and how my having HIV has affected them. I do a lot of beadwork and I don't want them touching any of my knives or needles. I tell them, "those things are mine just don't touch anything." It's another added stress when I have people come over and visit. I try to keep everything cleaned up, but it's hard, especially when I have to use a community kitchen and community bathrooms. The colds go around really fast.

I've been lucky so far this year, I haven't really gotten sick. I have been taking my meds for six months now; I take a lot of meds. In the morning, I take two tablespoons of a liquid, and during the day a handful of other pills. I used to be just on the AZT and T3s twice a day. Ray is on a different concoction than I am. I started drinking a few weeks ago and one of my daughters said, "Mom, I don't want you drinking." I don't want to hurt their feelings but yet I have to think of myself though.

The medicine I take is working, but day in, and day out you don't think you're doing anything, but it takes its toll. They had to invent these clear plastic pills because, before, it was like taking chalk, that really made your throat throb badly. It's like taking aspirins without the lining; you will get a really bad sore throat really fast.

Ray and I started taking the meds together and every three months we go in for blood work. He went from whatever and started getting better. This second time he went in, the virus was undetect-able; there's no trace of HIV in him anymore. My blood isn't doing so good but I think it's getting better. They really stress that if you don't follow the schedule, it'll go on reverse on you, instead of work-ing the other way, and exasperate it even faster.

I will be all right, as long as I am part of a study or group. I don't think they are taking any survey or study on women who are still abusing everyday and these pills they are taking; there is no study on that. I just wish that there would be a study of people like us. The pain is there and you've got to get rid of it. That is the only way that I can deal with it. Also, if I don't have my Gravol I end up throwing up all this stuff so it wouldn't work. And sleepers, if I don't have my sleepers, I don't sleep. It's just one drug to the next and the next and it does hurt.

There's an annual conference called, "Healing Our Spirits." I really think it is good. I went to the one that was in Nanaimo. My sister Irene was there, and when I saw her, I left. I just couldn't stay for the whole thing. There's just something about her when I see her,

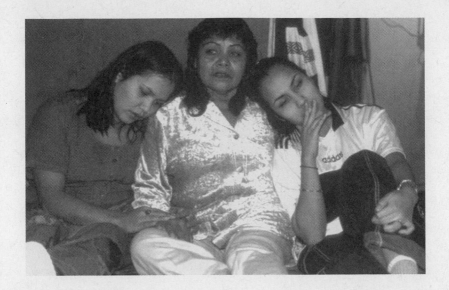

I think of bad things and I can't stand her. When I do talk to her she will pick up on the same argument wherever she was at before. She will say the same words, same tone; she will get right back into the same emotion that she was in. If it takes her ten years to finish an argument, then that's how long she will take. I can't do anything, I can't think and that is pretty sad. It is sad and it feels like I am passing that onto the kids. I know they all feel the same way about her as I do, but they just don't know how to explain it and they don't know why. I don't know why, but I know why it's just that I don't have no way of letting it out or explaining it without losing it all.

I think there are a lot of things out there that people are doing and it's good because a lot of work needs to be done. There is no one asking the people, especially the women that live with HIV and AIDS, what they think. I think we're the ones that are most abused, because the men don't want to use condoms and yet they still go out and screw around.

Neelum

SIMA QADEER

Neelum had been told that it took courage to be human. But, as she waited for the blow to fall on her mother's face, she wondered whether it was courage or fear that held her mother still, inert almost. She watched through curious detached eyes as first her mother's spine straightened, then, as her feet braced themselves on the floor, her body preparing itself for the impact of the fist being aimed at her left cheek. She wondered whether her mother was even aware of her body's response, it was so instinctive, like an animal. The blow came and, as mother's head snapped back from the pressure of meaty knuckles on bony cheek, Neelum slowly turned her head and vomited.

Neelum fought the dizzying rush of consciousness. A cracked eyelid revealed beams of weak winter sun on her duvet. Blocking out the light, Neelum pondered the merits of making today the day. Her brother was supposed to come into town later that night so he would be there to see her parents through the ordeal. She would time it so that her parents, her mother, wouldn't be alone for too long before he came in. The day ahead was free; her only appointment was with her psychiatrist. She could always cancel that. Now what should be the method? Neelum stretched and yawned. It had to be pain free. She had a very low threshold for pain. She never understood how people managed to take themselves out by hangings or gunshot wounds. Another overdose? The last one didn't work, so perhaps it was best to try another way, the running car in the garage? That would be nice. Painless. Neelum pulled the covers over her head and waited for the moment when Morpheus would take over again. The running car in the garage; she imagined it would be like going to sleep.

They keep on telling her that she should forget, that it had nothing to do with her, that it did not happen to her. She was not the victim they told her. Yet, like a photo album, she kept on seeing the images, turning them over in her mind. They are all that she would inherit. They were her legacy, proof that she had ever existed that she had ever experienced life. The pictures frequently blend together and she often forgot the date or the reason. Sometimes it would be because dinner was late, or was not warm enough. Other times it was because he had a bad day at work or he didn't have any clean clothes. But forever there, always constant, is that tiny desperate face with huge swollen eyes, watching quietly from the corner, watching the scene unfold, held transfixed by the moment. The pathetic little body breathes deeply, taking huge breaths into the starved body. The eyes watch with a combination of emotions, fear, horror, and curiosity. They ask her why she can't let it go. They don't understand. These pictures are hers.

They are all that she has to explain the twisted pain that lives inside her. Without those photos she wouldn't know, she would just think she was mad.

The psychiatrist would always start the sessions with the same questions. How was she doing? What was she thinking? She would pause and wonder how to answer him. Should she let him in? For her, the biggest problem with therapy was how intrusive it felt. Her thoughts were the one thing that she felt that she had ownership of, and she felt resentful of having to give that up. Would he understand? Whenever she spoke, she felt as if she was relaying anecdotes at a dinner party. It was as if the articulation of her feelings rendered them meaningless. Is each day a victory because she has survived? Or is it a testament to her failure as a human being? She felt that if she could make some sense of the madness, then she would have a purpose in living. How did her mother do it? Every time she looked at her mother it broke her. It wasn't so bad to be broken though. She felt it was better to be broken than to be whole and always failing. What did she want? A rebirth perhaps, to never have known of this existence. To never have been. To never have lived in this body, to never have seen this face, to never have used this mind. The ultimate freedom is to not exist at all. That is what she wished for. Not to die. Because death would mean that she had been. She wanted to never have been, to never have known anything of this girl Neelum. Should she tell him all this?

"I'm fine," she replies instead, and smiles. "I have been doing okay."

Promised Land

RANDA HAMMADIEH

They wrenched it violently from my shaking hand MY
stone, MY symbol.
Sirens screaming resounding in my skull,
gripping me and tearing into my innermost core,
flooding my entire being.
Where is my promised peace!
But I am entrenched in this land,
my roots as deep and extensive as those of the olive
tree,
whose bitter plant, now nurtured by the wailing blood-
soaked earth,
gives no sustenance.
My soul has been crucified,
upon the land which I cultivated,
upon the land where my innocence was shattered,
into a million pieces,
and curdled into cold black rocks
tempting me and beckoning to me wherever so I walk.

Hands that Care

NEETA SINGH

(Dedicated to Eslin Payne, who single-handedly runs
the Youth Centre, Hands That Care, in Toronto).

You created
your brainchild
Hands That Care
single-handedly
As a single mom
it is not just an agency
It is not just a Centre
It is the magic
in your hands
your healing touch
that is a constant;
it is not just the
Community-award
the $200-a-plate
Women of Distinction dinner
That you constantly overlook
it is your dignity,
your love, your aura
of motherliness, of passion
and drive
that we applaud
and hope will be passed
down several generations –
Let us continue
your efforts,
by word of mouth

Who says the oral tradition
does not exist?
We pray for your success
every night
for Eslin, you have
Hands That Care
and what you have created
in reality
Is you.

Enter the Lion's Den: A Journey to the Centre of My Uterus – One Black Woman's Story of Fibroids

WENDY VINCENT

When I left university and began working, I wore a size two in all of my clothing. As I became entrenched in the working world, this two gradually slipped into a four. I credited this to living downtown and eating out A LOT, and fitness wise, changing from jazzercise to a full-out gym membership with weights and a cardio routine.

The gym was my demon though; despite my bi-weekly membership fees, after some time, I fell out of my routine and I fell hard. We always hear about how gym attendance must be maintained and how quickly muscle turned to fat. When my belly began to grow, I immediately blamed it on not going to the gym, eating out, and eating late. There was more; everything from menstrual bloating to shrinking clothes. I had no idea that all the while, large, multiple fibroids had set in and had started to grow in my uterus.

I heard it all. Some of my tackier friends had asked me if I was pregnant. University friends commented on my weight gain. Family friends shrilled that I had finally put on weight and how it looked good. Another said, "don't go on a diet!" Just get back to the gym and tighten up those abs. A colleague mentioned how cute my little tummy was. As I struggled into and disguised myself in whatever items from my wardrobe that I had not thrown out in frustration and embarrassment, I continued to ignore my expanding but very centred girth. I felt guilt over wasted gym dues, I felt ashamed of my increasingly conspicuous belly.

All the while, my period remained as painful. If not, increasingly so. My pain threshold had surpassed the medication I had been prescribed and sought over the years. Again, I did not question it.

I only thought that it was my body just becoming immune to the medicinal alleviation. I was told that strong stomach muscles were a cure-all for bad cramps. I don't recall any relief during the best of my stomach crunches. I merely accepted that I was born to have a painful period. I recall so vividly the intense pain of my first period when I was twelve years old. I remember a distant comment by my mother, while laying on top of a hot water bottle, that her oldest sister always suffered with cramps. The missed classes throughout high school and university, and through to my working life. The increasing fatigue despite morning primrose, multivitamins plus iron, random meals with red meat, and increased food portions to compensate for my exercise routine. Meditation, reflexology, and chocolate were all flimsy bandages. Eventually I became dependent on some over-the-counter medication, which was not available in Canada, and which was always running dangerously low.

Even when I eventually began experiencing discomfort and soreness after my period, I had an answer. My stomach was retrocontracting. Relaxing itself after the pressure of my monthly menses, which weren't really monthly at all; given my size, my period was heavy and it came often. When I was planning my vacation to Africa, I put my foot down. This had to be regulated. I could, thanks to the drugs, take the pain like a man, but there was no way that I would be willing to suffer from random, heavy bleeding all the way at the other end of the earth. I had been caught with my pants down on vacation before, but this could be a nightmare. After a pap test, I got my prescription for Demulen. I menstruated for twenty-five days straight. The only thing *wrong* that I could surmise, after consulting with peers and my doctor, was that the prescription was merely too strong. So I switched.

The next prescription was fine and I was set for my trip. All this time I became increasingly aware of my stomach and how it just looked plain swollen. My ideal wardrobe for Africa and my usual summer clothes this year were going to be tight, unattractive, and uncomfortable. I made it through with my soon-to-be-uniform disguise of layers and lots of loose button downs. For the most part, I was tottering between a four and six with what looked like a really big gut. Nothing else was *growing* on me so I continued not to question anything.

My first recollection that something was really wrong was one night before bed when I decided to poke about and feel what was really going on with my belly. I touched and felt a tough knot in my stomach. I credited an unmetabolized meal to the mound. When I felt it again two nights later, I knew it was trouble. But how bad? Maybe tension about work and the trip. It was too close to me leaving, and though I was genuinely scared, I refused to have it checked out. If there was something terribly wrong, it would have to wait; this Black woman was going to Africa first. It was the last thought I ever gave to the situation.

As someone who ate out often, I now recall meals that would disappear for days as they struggled to metabolize in my obviously strained intestines

Despite heavy, frequent, painful periods, even random breakthrough bleeding, fatigue, constipation, a bloated stomach, and vague discomfort during sex, when I was having it, I suspected no single source for my various discomforts. I had been having checkups at the doctor and pap tests all this time. However, in early January, my situation came to a head.

After a week of intense discomfort, I had to find my way to the family doctor. Although that preternatural voice in the back of my head had been telling me to get my general medical situation in check, I had put it off for quite sometime. Despite moving out on my own downtown, I never made the doctor-change and, therefore, found myself commuting to the suburbs for my medical appointments. Instead of finding a more convenient doctor, the toil of this commute, of course, caused me to avoid going to the doctor whenever I *thought* I could.

As I mentioned, however, by the end of this particular bout of pain, I could not put it off any longer, and I was in fact lucky that this was one of the infrequent Saturdays that my doctor was open. I woke up early and called for the first available opening.

After being on the examination table for a while, the doctor felt my belly. He asked me if I needed to urinate, which I did. When

I was done, I hopped back onto the table. He nudged again. I was immediately informed that there was *something* in my womb; that I had the uterus of a woman who was five months pregnant.

Whatever it is, it's bad. It's either that you are pregnant or you have fibroids.

Poor bedside manners aside, I was shocked and immediately burst into silent tears. I had only been with my partner for three months, and the idea of being too pregnant to have choices, and for someone who did not love me, terrified me. Equally difficult to bear, upon hearing it was fibroids, was that I recall just days ago, my eldest cousin, the first woman born from my mother's generation, had a hysterectomy after her uterus could no longer bear the years of fibroids and the failure to reasonably combat them. What would be the outcome of this? I am a twenty-nine year old urban professional black woman who, for all intents and purposes, had every hope of using her uterus to have several children. Just not at this moment.

By the end of the weekend, and despite my doctor's insistence on a blood/pregnancy test, I was convinced that I was, indeed, not pregnant.

I spent the next two days reading up about fibroids. I had all of the symptoms. It was incredible. I never knew that they were related to one specific affliction. That heavy bleeding and constipation could be related seemed incomprehensible to me. I also read about the supposed causes and contributing factors. I was confused. Holistic practitioners mentioned poor diet in older than me black women, and the effects of having that poor diet accumulate within your digestive tract somehow. OB/GYN's in France cited red meat. I heard stress, chicken, estrogen, the pill, or not the pill, on Oprah, I heard that some women got fibroids because they were particularly preoccupied and worried about a particular situation in their lives. I am an assertively health-conscious eater and a woman under thirty. None of this applied to me and I felt as though I was reading something written in another language. Maybe I really was pregnant. The only remote linkage I could refer to was my recently *hysterectomized* cousin.

When the results confirmed that I was not with child, my next step was to have an ultrasound. After telling my partner about my situation, and getting the all clear on my pregnancy test, I told my parents about what was happening to me. While I spoke to my mother on the phone, she said the words which I will never, as long as I live, ever forget. "When I was your age, I had a fibroid the size of a grapefruit removed." Just like that. My own mother. Who sat eating her vegetables while we talked about Cousin Fanny's fibroids and resultant hysterectomy. What then becomes a blur to me is the instant when she told me that, not only did she have an overgrown, benign tumour cut from her uterus when she was pregnant with my brother, but also that of her five sisters, four of them had had fibroids removed. My mother, her sisters, my aunts. Twenty-nine years and I had no idea.

I soon reread one of the passages from some of the foreign-looking literature about fibroids. There it was in black and in white. Several generations of women from the same family are known and documented to have the disease.

I was completely devastated. Why had I not been told? What sort of legacy of ill-health and ignorance was I born into? Despite all the maternal and familial love in my life, at that moment I felt as though I were swimming in a pool of sharks. If only I had known.

A few days later, I received my ultrasound results. As it turns out, I had multiple fibroids, and they were large. My uterus is distended by five times the normal size in order to accommodate the tumours. All the years of wrenching cramps, the exhaustion, all of it. Cold comfort; my mother informed me that one of my aunts also had multiple fibroids.

I spent hours sitting by my window. Bitter at not being told. Bitter at having my uterus attacked. Bitter at facing the possibility of having my stomach cut open to free my womb from it's invaders.

It has now been three months since my initial diagnosis. To date I have not received any medical care. There have been weeks and weeks of test and impending results. The current selection of African-American women's magazines have recently published articles about sisters and fibroids: A woman cited in one magazine [ESSENCE], actually bled out her orange-sized fibroid at work one day after months of drinking chlorophyll and wearing a magnet on her stomach. In these publications, I also learned that phytoestrogens, found in soy product, are a combatant against the errant estrogen that is responsible for fibroids. My kitchen cupboards are now stocked with soy-protein-based foods.

Between my GP in Scarborough, a new doctor at the women's health clinic downtown, a new OB/GYN at Toronto General, and a scheduled surgeon consultation at Mount Sinai, this fibroid inflicted, child-bearing years, single black woman will eventually be seen to. In the meantime, I am eating as much tofu and soybean snacks as possible.

Women's Health in Scary Hands

KRISTINE MAITLAND

Two years ago I made the decision to have the hysterectomy. For me, it was the choice between screaming in pain for two-and-a-half weeks out of each month and not dealing with the stress of suffering. The latter choice was preferable.

I knew about all the *alternatives* (thanks to Oprah); indeed, I've tried many of them, including having a failed myomectomy. Doubly failed because, not only did the myomectomy not work, I was subjected to the incompetence of Canada-trained white nurses. Give me a forty-year old UWI (University of the West Indies) nurse any day. They, at least, can find a vein. As it was, I spent half an hour lying on an operating table, arms outstretched like a Black female Christ. And after half an hour of being stabbed in both arms, the surgeon herself managed to stick the IV in. A spear in the side would have been preferable.

You would think that I would avoid subjecting myself to the torture of the medical care system again. However, the economy being what it is, I did not have the luxury to "wait and see". Ultimately, it was either to have the pain stop and keep my job, or struggle some more and be out of a job due to all my absences.

As it happened, having the surgery was the easy part. It was the aftermath that proved to be the more hellish. At the hospital, my floor seemed to be staffed by unsupervised nursing students who, poor dears, didn't have a clue. As it was, I only saw a real nurse at night. A blond white woman in her forties, she was the one who handed me the sleeping pills, my only defence against the screaming patients on my floor.

Thank God I'm from a family of nurses. Two of my aunts came in to "special" for me. (*Specialing* means doing medical care short of actually dispensing medicines: Won't do to get sued, don't you know). It was my aunts who bathed me and helped me to the bathroom. My fellow inmates looked at me in envy. The nurses in my ward looked to me with relief. I was one less person that they had to deal with. Thinking on it now, it occurs to me that nobody at the hospital questioned the qualifications of my aunts. I guess the sight of West Indian women changing bed sheets and cleaning bedpans is an acceptable norm.

A machine provided my pain medication. Apparently, these drug vending machines are there to replace a (Black? Philippino?) nurse. Thanks, but no thanks. After two days of being completely stoned, I decided to go off the painkillers. I didn't think that being high was conducive to getting better.

On the morning of the third day, a student nurse gleefully removed the staples from my 210-pound stomach. One of my Aunts arrived just as the last staple came out. She sighed and rolled her eyes, like an obeah foreseeing the future. I was discharged from hospital. But the staples had been pulled out too soon and, needless to say, my wound split open the minute I got home. By 10:30 P.M., I was back at the hospital accompanied by my aunt, who had come from work to escort me back to the emergency room. I waited for two hours for a doctor to come and see me.

I was in the bathroom when he arrived so he said that he would come back later. My aunt, knowing that it could be another two hours before we saw him again (been there, seen that), begged and then, frustrated, yelled at him to stay. By the time I was on the table the doctor, who was a jerk to start with, and my aunt, were at each other's throats. It was I, split open as I was on the operating table, who had to act as peacemaker. "Uh, hello. I hate to interrupt this discussion, but my guts are starting to spill out onto the floor...."

Later on, two female doctors arrived, packed my belly, and sent me home with a bottle of saline, saying that a home care nurse would see me in the morning. I, of course, knew better: tomorrow was Good Friday. I was a former Catholic and was well aware of the fact that no help would be coming. When the doctors left, my aunt proceeded to swipe some gauze from the room. "Count on these doctors to think that we have this stuff lying about at home." It is scary to think that in Ontario, sick people to have to resort to thievery. So much for "Oh help."

Ten years ago I would have said that I was treated badly because I was Black. But I know better – I live in Ontario, where all patients earning less than $50,000 a year are treated like crap.

So, after that, it was six weeks of home *scare* – which is the only way to describe the so-called home care I received. Every day I was visited by a stressed-out white nurse: she was seeing, on average, fifteen patients a day. It was she who had my mother boil my bandages, as well as the one pair of supposedly disposable forceps that could be spared. You would think that we lived in a third-world country. My mother, a former nurse, hadn't had to boil bandages since she had left the West Indies in the sixties.

Needless to say, I survived. Am I sorry for having had a hysterectomy? Hell no. Estrogen via hypodermic isn't that bad when you're only thirty years old. The loss of my reproductive organs has made me better appreciate the cranky infant and the terrible toddler. But this experience is also taught me the responsibility that can be brought to bear on an *auntie*, and I wear the badge of *auntie* with pride.

Morí Soñando / I Died In My Dreams

INGRID RIVERA

En mís sueños me muero
En mís sueños me muero

Acostada en la felicidad
Flotando en la corriente de azúcar moreno
Una rebanada de flan lista para ser devorada – (en realidad)
Pero la muerte ya no es una opcíon
No puede ser
No debe ser

Morí soñando
En mí cuarto –color de pasteles – (marrón)

Oscuro y solitario
Oliendo la muerte de mi corazón
Parecido a un pimiento pegado al fuego
Asfixiada como un pedazo de carne
Profunda en el horno
(de mami)

Papi
Sordo
Sus orejas cortadas
y tiradas en el agua hervida

Morí soñando
En mí cuarto – color de pasteles – (marrón)

Lo sentí
Lo sentí otra vez
El sentido del dolor – confusión

Una gallina corriendo, corriendo y corriendo sin cabeza –
    decapitada
Un dolor tan profundo que lo siento en mí alma
Agitada por la corrida
Quisiera caerme
Deseo liberarme
de lastima

Colocada en el medio de la mesa
Dejando cada uno tomar un pedazo de mí
realidad
Consumiendolo
Desapareciendo
Hasta que mí cuerpo – mís pensamientos, no existen más
Deshacerme de este dolor
Quedandome en paz

Ansiedad de retirar lo que no puedo cambiar....
Todavia la agonía me posee
Pesar, confusión, miedo y estupidez

Morí soñando
En mí cuarto

Marrón
Oscuro
Ciega
Sigo con el sueño
El sueño
Un sueño

Morí soñando
Sigo con el deseo
El deseo
Un deseo

Deseo de morir – pero no soñando (en mis sueños)

In my dreams I die
In my dreams I die

Laying in happiness
Floating in the current of brown sugar
A slice of crème caramel ready to be devoured – (in reality)
But death is no longer an option
It can't be
It shouldn't be

I died in my dreams
In my room – the colour of *pasteles* – (brown)

Dark and lonely
Smelling the death of my heart
Resembling a pepper set on fire
Suffocated like a slab of meat
Deep in my mother's oven
Dad – deaf
Ears chopped off and thrown into boiling water

I died in my dreams
In my room – the colour of *pasteles*– (brown)

I felt it
I felt it again
The feeling of hurt – confusion

A chicken running and running and running with her head cut off
    – decapitated
A pain so deep I feel it in my soul
Agitated from the run
I want to fall
I wish to rid myself of this hurt

Placed in the centre of the table
Letting each one take a piece of my reality
Consuming it
Making it disappear
Until my body – my thoughts, no longer exist
Ridding myself of this pain
To be in peace

Yearning to take back what cannot be changed
Still the agony possesses me
Regret, confusion, fear, and stupidity

I died in my dreams
In my room

Brown
Dark
Blind
The dream continues
The dream
A dream

I died in my dreams
The desire continues
The desire
A desire

Desire to die – but no longer in my dreams

Oh My Aching Feet

NORA BURRELL

For years I have had problem feet. At first it was just one foot, but as the years move on, the two of them decide to work together. Sometimes my feet itch, sometimes they burn, and sometimes they even bite. You know, I sit now and I'm afraid to get up, because the cramping may start. I can't wear certain shoes because they are so swollen. I went to the doctors so often, I even say to myself, one day they will get tired of me. The doctors gave me ointment to anoint them, they told me, when I sit down I should put them up. I did everything I was told to do. I used home remedies. Sometimes they feel tight. I prayed to God, asking him to heal me. All my life I've lived with aching feet. I have days when my feet give me a break. I start getting dressed to go to work; putting on my shoes is a problem because my heel back is feeling sore. So I can't wear the shoes I was putting on, and I wore those same shoes yesterday. Sometimes I wonder if they will ever get better. I wish the day would come when I can wear the shoes I like. My ankle feels like I have a rubber band around it, my knee cap is so stiff; I have to drag them. I said, oh God, please give me the strength to go on. Oh my aching feet, what would I do without them.

ethnic ph.d.

BELDAN SEZEN

the name is b./ i don't want to be pushed/ i don't want to be named/ i don't want to be crushed/ i don't want to be tamed/ no matter who you are/ do not try to fix me/ any kind of stagnation is death/ italk what ic, iwalk what ib.

ethnic ph.d.

no no no-ho
not
      gonna be
your
      ethnic ph.d.

no no no-ho
not
      gonna be
your
      ethnic research-e

no no no-ho

for you
>
> I don't want to develop

my

>
> intellectuality

>
> don't want to discover

my

>
> sexuality

>
> don't want to analyse

my

>
> reality

to fulfill the picture in

>
> your fantasy

no no no-ho
not

>
> gonna be

your

>
> ethnic ph.d.

thin line

BELDAN SEZEN

(respect 2 Kid Frost)

"it's a thin line between love and hate
it's a thin line between love and hate"

inside me
there is a thin line
that makes me love
that makes me hate
hate myself
love myself
a thin line
between love and hate

ain't no white
ain't no beautiful
and i never can be
as white and beautiful as you want
to make me
belive
i shall be
but when i look at you
i ain't see no beauty
just cold eyes
and ugly faces
"it's a thin line between love and hate
it's a thin line between love and hate"

inside me
there is a thin line
that makes me love
that makes me hate
hate myself
love myself
a thin line
between love and hate

ain't no white
ain't no beautiful
and i never can be
as white and beautiful as you want
to make me
believe
i shall be
but when i look at you
i ain't see no beauty
just cold eyes
and ugly faces
ain't no space for beauty
inside me
just this thin line
can't be white and beautiful
just want to be me
it's a lie
that you try
to make me swallow
can't love a lie
can't live a lie
ain't not me
what i see
want to be me
and still:
"it's a thin line between love and hate"

I Crawl into Earth

VERA WABEGIJIG

i

Dig my fingers deep
Into moist dark earth I burrow
A hole big enough to crawl into,
Go back where I came from,
Into my mother's belly.

ii

I never asked for life
not into this hell
of political shame
where spirits shy away from

this place called life
a place of hunters and gatherers
where vampire hunters
gather us together just to suck
our energy and seize our spirit

in this land, so vast with resources
from this sacred earth
no one should go hungry
or go without shelter
yet, my brothers
and my sisters
are looked upon without compassion
without understanding hardship
or despair.

instead, we divert our eyes
and our eyes never meet
they deserve to be there
they want to be there
those street rats, skids
winos, crack heads
prostitutes, and pimps
and here we are sucking them dead.

in this city lie
full of concrete giants
that hover above our tiny bodies
like towering prison guards
blocking our escape
from manipulated dreams
of conquered nations, people

indians killed during a relay of false truths,
treaties signed with alcohol, false trades promoting
a partnership of land and shared resources,
building great civilized,
colonized nations
under one god who saves
savage indian souls

iii

my hole is dug deep
I crawl into it, the earth
my mother and I lie still
in this warm, dark womb
wrap my arms tightly around my knees
and hold them close to my chest
cradle the inner thunder that waits to strike
and tears like rain stream down down mountains
my body shakes, convulses
contractions tremble creation.

a full moon rises above me
a spotlight that protects
with nokimis giiziis medicine
her light cleanses the black
inside and outside of me
hush nadonis, her heart beats lullabies
urging me into dream
my body takes fetal shape

as the sun dances in the eastern sky
my eyes open, fluttering like a butterfly
I stretch stiff limbs
and on all ours like muskwa
I crawl out of earth, my mother, brand new.

GLOSSARY:
nokimis giiziis: moon; nadonis: daughter; muskwa: bear

Untitled

MARISA MAHARAJ

Salt water drips of my lips stepping out of the ocean
this ocean
this ocean and these waves
that lap and pull at my body like I'm chocolate milk
sweet and frothy, to be sucked up and digested
salt water cleanses and dries out my brown clothes
turns them darker and scarier and glowing
and beautiful
in this ocean I can't survive
it surrounds too much, leaves too much space
and too little time for movement, for swimming
especially for me....
I'm left always standing in the ocean
too many ways to go
too many waves to drag me around
when the shores are constantly distant

Spake Ginty Spake

ANAKANA SCHOFIELD

The net curtains inside the van were lifted and just as quickly flattened, pressed by sturdy fingers into the corners of the van windows, as the small, red Fiat Uno with its radio tuned to Planet FM, cruised over the potholed lane that led up to the collection of caravans gathered together on the halting site.

It was extraordinary, the stillness in the site as Sarah Connor put the car in neutral, pulled the handbrake up, and heard the radio click out as she pulled the keys from the ignition. Every time she'd previously visited, the site had been bustling with activity.

She reached into the back seat and lifted a black file folder. Her hand touched the Marks and Sparks bag that contained her Potato-au-gratin ready-made dinner. She was psyched. This was one of a many visits into this community. She'd followed the advice and guidance of her mentor at University College Dublin. She was ready.

"First you go in and win the community's trust, and then you get them to speak. Don't expect to get much the first few visits." The prof had told her.

She'd been patient, warm, enthusiastic, and not too pushy.

"Then you stop being so polite about it, and by then, you have their trust and they should open up like tulips and provide all imaginable information."

Today was her last attempt to visit; she needed to make progress on the questionnaires contained in her file. She had gotten quite a bit of info on the last visits, but today's stuff was more sensitive.

Two areas in particular, she'd got no movement from these women. Health and domestic violence. It was touchy, but she had to get someone talking. It was tough asking a woman whether her menstrual cycles were regular, if she took the pill, did she smoke, drink, consume coca cola, take regular exercise, when she knew the community had neither electricity nor running water.

She had done her research:

"Travellers are a small, indigenous minority, documented as being part of Irish society for centuries. The distinctive Traveller lifestyle and culture is based on a nomadic tradition.... Only 5 per cent of Travellers live to be fifty years old."

"Travellers have different perceptions on health," she'd read specifically on the more difficult topics.... *"They may experience problems engaging the services of doctors."*

She'd read every thesis written about Travellers. She'd devoured two studies only last night on the representation of travellers in the media. By the end of them she had felt fired up over inequality.

She found statements like: *"... The court was right to note the extent of the discrimination and prejudice experienced by Irish Travellers...."*

"... Traveller infant mortality is three times greater than the national average,"

"... Traveller women have a life expectancy of sixty-five years," floating through her brain, the way a person might read the back of a cereal packet and find the ingredients circling their brain for days on end.

She was different, she was indeed. Sure, only last week when she'd been home for the weekend to Kildare, she'd tackled her younger brother Ronán with the tactics of a Welsh rugby player. She smiled thinking about the exchange,

- *"There's no Traveller wedding, funeral, or baptism in this country where there isn't blood spilt by those people,"* he started proclaiming loudly when she told him of her study.

She recognized the proclamation instantly; their father had often held forth in the same manner.

- *"Ah here, not a single one,"* she prodded him. *"There must be one, or have you cameras recording what happens at every single one. You're absolutely certain about that now? Because …"*

He'd said nothing; she could tell he felt stupid. She let his stupidity sit in the air for a few seconds before launching into him.

- *"What about the young fella killed last month, the fella who died under the wheels of a bus being kicked to death by a bunch of fellas your age, and them all watching and all. That was no Traveller wedding, funeral, or baptism,"* she told him straight, *" that was just a regular old Saturday night disco in these parts with idiot young fellas like yourself. The Four Courts are full of cases."*

Her brother had continued muttering into his greasy fringe.

- *"I suppose you'd say similar things about asylum seekers too?"* she jibed him. *"I suppose it's only them too who are responsible for every bad feckin thing that happens in this Godforsaken country."*
- *"Sure, they all have mobile phones,"* was his reply.
- *"Of course they do, sure, don't they need them for avoiding the likes of you. They're probably calling each other up warning themselves when they see you approach. Racist white idiot moving down O'Connell St, he's on the bridge, oh no, the big Gom is on his way toward me. The government should supply them with them free to help them navigate some of the pathetic eejits they have to deal with."*

She'd stood up and left the room. Let him think about that. She expected more of him.

This evening she felt proud that she'd tackled him, as she turned the telly on to watch Coronation Street. She fell asleep as Rita Fairclough was pulling her milk bottles in off the street.

Driving to the halting site the next morning in her dad's car, she felt an affinity to the Travellers, like she understood them (after all she'd read so much about them), she was connected to them.

A few roads before she pulled into the site, she felt an urgency. Today she needed their co-operation. Together they could triumph over inequality. I may even keep coming out here to visit them once it's done, she thought, in a warm moment, she imagined a friendship brewing between them all.

The more pressing reason for getting fired up over inequality and discrimination against Travellers was the looming prospect she'd have to face her professor in a one-on-one meeting at the end of the week. She needed to gather all her interviews and pull some conclusions from them. She needed to collate the statistics available, with the results of her own study. (This project had a deadline and she intended to meet it.)

Around the same time Rita Fairclough had been pulling milk bottles off the street on Coronation Street, Ginty gathered the women in the halting site telling them straight:

- *"I'm getting fierce tired of all the questions going on around here."*

She didn't mention the student girl by name, but the girls knew who it was she meant. She was the only persistent settled visitor of late.

- *"We're only encouraging the likes of her,"* she told them; her foot resting on an *auld* stone at the bottom of the few steps that led up to her caravan.

The girls had all nodded at her.

- "*An' I want no mention of me, do ya hear? I'm not here if any of them asks. I don't have anything to say to the likes of her. They're always after me to say a few words about this and that. I've no words left for them.*"

It was widely acknowledged that Ginty had once been a spokesperson on behalf of all Travellers. For a few years, whenever a story broke about Travellers, the national TV station would wheel her out to give a few comments on the six o'clock news. Even the morning radio shows wanted to interview her. It was strange the way they ran out of time, if she said anything other than answer the question they asked her. Say, if she began to expand on a point, there was never any time for it. Seeing how nothing had changed for Travellers, Ginty got plain pissed off and refused to ever give another comment again, even if the Pope came banging at her caravan door.

The women were used to people not being here; since feuds did happen and people sometimes had to keep a low profile.

They were fluent enough at saying

- "*He's not here. I've not seen him.*" Now, they simply had to switch the him, with a her.

Rumour had it that Ginty's husband was himself killed years back because of a feud with another family. Since Ginty wouldn't utter a word on the subject, it was only speculation. It was no beggar's business. It was never anyone's business when the talk was about your husband.

After losing her husband, Ginty had turned her attention to music. She was a great lover of song and music. She had enormous expense keeping her radio in batteries since she ran it day and night. The whole community had a barometer on her state of mind, depending which way the radio was tuned.

Sarah Connor stepped out of her dad's car, running through the questions and techniques she might use this morning. I don't want to make you feel uncomfortable but.... How do you feel about.... I understand that these issues may stir sensitive emotions in you....

It all sounded so official and sterile. A moment flickered where, for a coupling of seconds, she wished, for her own sake and the sake of these women, she did not have to through the rigmarole. These mere seconds gave rise to a bay-window-sized thought; was anything really going to be changed on account of these interviews and the conclusions she would draw and present to her mentor? These thoughts slowed her initially confident strides towards the first door on which she intended to knock.

Rapping assertively on the first door, the sound of her knuckles reverberated and she found her repeated knocks were not of the same fortitude.

She'd approached three caravans and as she'd knocked more questions pounded her.

Her knocking had gotten lighter and lighter to the point where she noticed her knuckles were no longer making contact with the door at all. Her wrist was making a fluttering motion and that was all.

Her head was rattling.

Would anyone ever read this study of hers? She was only a social science student. She had no official capacity to be assessing anyone or the like. Did she have any real interest in this kind of work at all?

She began to admit to herself that the situation for Travellers was brutal in Ireland, that prejudice was stacked against them. They'd sort of fallen into her lap as a project. Now she found herself reducing the enormity of their problems and struggles to a heap of yellow post-it notes and a decent project mark.

The most critical thing that could come from all of this was she might go up in the opinion of her important, but grumpy professor. This was the way it was out there with student fieldwork.

Could you bring back a startling quote, a good statistic? Could you reduce the most unacknowledged social problem to an interesting bunch of sentences with your name at the top?

After the third caravan, she'd had enough of the rattling going round her head; she had all the information she needed. She'd take these thoughts back and commit them to paper.

She began to retreat towards the red Fiat when a yodeling shriek emitted from underneath the gap of the door and through the small windows of the fourth caravan along in the group of fourteen.

One
      day
            at a time
                  sweet Jesus...."

Ginty let out a yowl that was off the piano scale altogether.

Tomorrow
      may
            never
                  be mine...."

An almost Aretha-Franklin-inspired harmony followed as the door was flung wide and Ginty flew down the steps clutching a teapot, singing into the distance as she spun round the van, swinging the pot over her head, releasing its contents all over the muck.

Sarah Connor took a few steps gingerly toward her. Then retreated.

By Euston Station she sat down.

ANAKANA SCHOFIELD

she awakes to the scars and haze
in the thinness of his skin
seams unravel
as swift as the smell of cheap sherry
would knock a pig

     his eyes roll back in his head laughing

       "I'm in a bit of trouble, like you, you know,"

sitting by her on a fountain in Euston Station he sounds like her
   uncle

how grey the day is
so grey
the sky could spit urine on them

      he laughs again

Mary wanders up clutching a half-filled bottle of port
same brand she shares it nimbly
offering our Girl Friday a sip

things haven't got that bad but she's heading there

"I've always hated nurses," he says
"Ireland produced a nation of nurses and I hate every one of them."

sherry sprinkles from his lips at the word nurses
his tongue chases it

"They're a bunch of bastarding bitches," Mary hiccups

"Why don't you go home to Ireland," Girl Friday asks them

"Nothing for me there, nothing for me here,"

sounds like a Judy Garland song
sung against the backdrop of a waterless fountain
drenched in pigeon shit, empty chocolate wrappers lie
untreated bi-polar disorder floats.

on her way to the arches she sees a tent
middle of a main road
drills reverberate into unprotected ears
guts tumble roadward sadly
no longing to be hoisted

the population of this temporary tarpaulin town consumes
enough grease to clog a nations heart
for breakfast
        they'll provide
Macadam under noble feet.

by afternoon our Girl Friday has wandered to the arches at
   London's Waterloo Station
she finds more members of her tribe
as they pause between sherry grunts and gasps
she recognizes their accents as Irish as her own

our Girl Friday has a home
she can't go to since
her neighbour threatened to kill her

the trouble started the very day after
her Jamaican fella put his head
down on the pillow by hers

a peaceful head
      snoozing

            consternation exploded up and down the stairs of
            that cheapshit building

she took to the streets the morning after
he lay his head
scooped them into
her palm

she wanders
sees the fate her people have met
whilst she typed a million memos
signed by men named Michael

"*Life shows you where you're headed,*" she thinks

centuries of nights spent
in front of the telly
drinking Pepsi
listening to drone of grim northern
soap operas
where folks fill pubs at lunchtime
then leave

have given her cottonwool brain

eating cheap meat
with no-think gravy
instead of cheap drink

She may not be drinking from the same bottle
yet she understands their lifting

the innocent seams of ignorance
have split

My People Paid

SHIRLEY BROZZO

In 1492
Columbus sailed the ocean blue
Wind filled the sails
Maps were askew
He thought he'd found India
Named us anew

And my people
Paid
With our blood

In 1607
Jamestown was born
Colonists were starving
Powhatan gave them some corn
They survived
They thrived
No longer to mourn

And my people
Paid
With our honour

Louisiana Purchase
Treks to the west
Further they pushed us
Further removed
Taking the land that was best
Pushed us and moved us
Moved us and pushed
Towards the ocean
The mountains
The badlands
And just

My people
Paid
With our land

Hollywood images
Mascots galore
Whopping
Face painting
Dancing on gym floors
Took our self-esteem
Self-worth
Pride
And more

And my people
Paid
With self-respect

It's 2002
Time for change is here
Stand up and speak
Raise a voice
Strong and clear
Our religion
Culture
Language
Now strong
Time for change
Is here

As my people
Reclaim
our lives!

The Circle of Life

PITCHE WASAYANANUNG

The seed stayed, waiting, waiting patiently, listening, sensing, exploring outwardly "I am so very thirsty, for one drop of water I would be so grateful. I am so afraid I will shrivel up and disappear altogether. Oh, what's that," listening intently drip, drop, drip, drop, seed is starting to feel so anxious and excited, the soil is starting to get wet, moist, the little seed is starting to move very slowly, reaching upwards to that now ever-increasing moistness. As seed did this, her tiny shell started to slowly crack. The crack got bigger as she continued to stretch towards the moisture; slowly from within this crack, appeared a tiny wisp of green. The green peeped through the top of the crack. "Hello." The green wisp started to stretch towards the moisture too, taking in a very big drink of delicious rain saying "YUM." Little green wisp sprung upwards at such a speed, that … the next moment little green wisp was blinded by a very bright yellow light. "OH." The light hurt, yet felt good at the same time, "MY, OH MY;" little green wisp found herself stretching her long green arms outwards and upwards. Arms that little green wisp did not know she even had, "WELL." Next, from within, little green wisp felt something growing upwards, "OH, OH," a bud burst out from little green wisp to form her head, "WOW, that felt good." Bud looked around at brightness filled with wonderful smells and sights, many other buds just like herself stood nearby, all waving their slender green arms at her, "WELCOME," they echoed in unison. Before little bud could respond to their kindness, she felt a quivering within her budness, "AGAIN." Very slowly she felt herself open upwards and outwards in all directions. Then, from somewhere, she heard, BUZZZ, BUZZZ. "What's that?" Then something landed on top of her causing her to giggle. "You're the most beautiful-smelling flower I have ever landed on," came a voice.

"I'm a flower?"

"A beautiful purple flower."

"Oh my ... what are you doing?"

"I'm taking nectar, to make honey for food for us bees."

"Oh."

So, little seed had many, many more adventures, meeting other wonderful and interesting life forms, yet that's another story.

My Room of Silence

ROLANDA KANE

My room silence is my circle of peace.
My centre of hope, my guidance of life.
Like the wind in the rain, like the footprints
in the sand. My room of silence is my window
of peace.

Mother's Prayer

ROLANDA KANE

In loving memory of my mother
Mrs. Madeline Suella Kane.

For the women and children all over the world, that labour
with the hopes of having just a little of their hard earnings for
themselves at the end of their workday, these words are for you.

Come my child sit talk with me?
Come my child share a little of your deepest thoughts with me.
I ask not that you kneel,
I ask not that you stand,
only the soft sweet words of your whispers grace this peaceful land.
You see there is a wonderful world of magic that stand as grace for
    us,
so today let us take a minute and feel its wonders amongst us.
Let the wind speak our voices,
let the sands shape our hands,
let the shadows of two worlds in passing
for today a mother and child shall pray.
Come my child sit and talk with me?
Come let me share a little of my deepest thoughts with you, for
    today is our day.
I ask not that you kneel, I ask not that you stand. Let heaven and
    earth find its
place with us for this day a mother and child shall make their
    stand.

Come my child sit and talk with me?
Come my child share just a little of your passing spirit, as it grows
   and pass its
living through you to me. Come my child, come share your prayers
   with me,
lie (take rest) upon a mother's wings in prayer.

Amen

This Body of Mine

ROLANDA KANE

April 6, 1996
Tshelanyemba, Zimbabwe

It is only through the timetable of our living
that the body of our forgiveness has once again opened its eyes.
Somewhere between body and mind it has lifted its head to give
    name
to the nameless.
Once upon a lifetime the balance of two worlds buried deep within
    the ashes
of our ancestral freedom lies its mystery, the inherited.
The ancient oneness hidden somewhere between the centre of what
    we have
yet to find.
Awaken its spirit to forth come and take its stand beside the ancient
    ritual.
The rebirth of its soul.

Gitane's Voice

GITANE WILLIAMS

In July 2000, I turned the young age of forty. For the most part, I have been blessed with great health in mind, body, and spirit. From my experience of being in a black female body, my weight has mostly been a battle – up some years and down others – but this has never been a health issue for me.

At the age of sixteen, I had my first memorable experience with the western medical model. During that year, I was complaining that my knees were bothering me. My mother took me to the children's hospital in Oakland, California, where I am a native of the Bay Area.

My knees were being overworked from playing sports year-round in school, and my overweight was the obvious reason. After many doctors, they really didn't know, so I ended up having an exploratory operation.

This was the end of my faith in medical models and the beginning of seeking alternative methods of healing. This journey has taken me to a mind/body connection – i.e. God is the first source of faith and healing – then to acupuncture, as a modality. I was healed and returned to my life without any reservation. Was this real? For me it was, and I lived healthy in my body for many years.

On or about the age of twenty-one to twenty-three, I was having what I now know as ulcers. This seemed familiar because a lot of my female black friends and family, including my mother, seemed to be under a lifestyle of stress, and it manifested in areas of lower intestine tract. Is this common?

My symptoms included ache, inability to keep food in the body, loss of water, etc. This went on for a while because, really, who could go to the doctors or who had insurance? Therefore, I was forced to go to the local clinics.

In this case it was West Oakland Medical Clinic. All right here it is.... After seeing the doctor, and whoever, they told me again that it was my diet, my lifestyle, my fault, or at least my responsibility to take care of myself. I was given the prescription; it was for an antacid – Midol. But, since my ulcer was eating me up so fast, I was told to drink half-and-half milk every thirty minutes, before taking the Midol, every four hours to smother the ulcer. Now, this is the finale for me.... I was kind of standing and leaning over with pain when I happen to look up! All I saw was shelves of the blue bottle all over the pharmacy, nothing else. There were now one standing in the back, filling bottles with pills, no other type of medication in sight, nothing but that blue bottle. Then I looked up and noticed all the black people waiting in line to get their meds. This was the moment I knew that my body was not open to being on any assembly line of treatment. I also knew that I had to get control over my life ... and recreate it another way. Yes, I did take the medication, and soon changed my life forever around diets, medication, and creating a stress-free environment for myself.

This is one example of what I've been exposed to and when I've chosen to do something differently about my health. As I mentioned before, I still have more questions, Sophie, than answers. I pray that all my health needs will come to me. What I am working with now is why is it that black women seem to have fibroids? At least five women in my community have had or have heavy bleeding and need to get some sort of treatment. Including me. The beat goes on....

Ode to Marie

ANA BODNAR

There is a woman I know. She comes to my office almost every week. She has been coming for over two years. She used to hit her kids. Very badly. Threw the eldest against the wall violently. She couldn't stop. She had been raped for years. This boy came from one of the rapes. Now he is ten and lives in a treatment centre. For now, maybe, not forever. He has tantrums and seizures. He has to be sat upon, his hands pulled back, in order for him to stop. This woman visits her son, every week, sometimes twice a week. She goes with her married lover, who will probably leave her in a year or so, like all of the others. Her son screams and yells and falls into a tantrum when his mother gets ready to leave. She doesn't understand how her boy could love her after all she did to him. She finds her actions unforgivable. She believes that she is detestable for hitting and kicking and screaming and maybe worse. I tell her, try to tell her, that when a child is hurt, he or she will make an even greater bond. The fear and the pain make a bond of intensity, a bond of trauma. A bond that is like a sliver of light in a tunnel of darkness. And this sliver of light is visited and held and clung to. And it is this sliver that provides the food for anything to grow and live. For the heart to stay a real heart, and not turn to glass or mush or swamp. So, this sliver is but a small fraction of the realms and seas and skies and trees and jewels that exist and have always existed. But when you are small, and all you see is up and down, and not really too far at that, and all you know is that sliver, you think you are going to drop dead on the spot without a breath of that air. So you scream and yell when the one who threw you against the wall prepares to leave.

At least she is yours.

Learning with the Women: My Travels in First Nations Country

ANA BODNAR

In the ten years I have worked in First Nations communities and agencies all over Ontario, I have met women who have been my teachers and continue to be my teachers.

In many First Nations traditions, it is the women who are the keepers of the cultural teachings and who are the harbingers of change. It is they who begin the process of movement from the old to the new. Women are honoured in their many roles within the life cycle: women as elders, mothers, children, sisters, friends, and mothers of the earth. It is also the women who sometimes know suffering up close and personal.

Margaret, Cynthia, Linda, Mary, Lillian,[1] and other First Nations women were my teachers, my colleagues, my clients. There have been many women of the First Nations communities who have taught with me, learned with me, and with whom I have shared time in healing circles, counselling sessions, and conversations; in airplanes, coffee shops, and even in the sweat lodge.

It is in these many conversations that the women have taught me about love, about commitment, about justice, about just hanging in when things get tough. One of the greatest gifts that I received was the gift of humour. And the lesson of keeping the humour flowing in the midst of extremely difficult situations.

I am a woman of the European tradition, a psychologist brought in to assist professional staff, community groups, and individuals in dealing with the immense grief and bereavement related to the suicide crisis that still continues in northwestern Ontario. This crisis has claimed the lives of young people, sometimes children as young as eleven years of age. Although there have been many programs aimed at reducing the suicide crisis in northwestern Ontario, suicide continues to be a serious problem.

My own particular role was to assist the project by bringing Western psychological concepts and tools and exploring how we might integrate traditional First Nations and Western tools and concepts. Based in northwestern Ontario, our work was intended to help communities and individuals mourn the loss of their youth to suicide. The statistics are staggering: First Nations youth have a suicide rate eight times higher than the national average.

My involvement was intensive, consisting of some twenty trips north over the period of two years, staying one week each time. I loved this work. It allowed me to use many different skills, develop new talents, and work with interesting and diverse team members. My role was to train staff, carry out psychological assessments, and provide counselling, while also doing community-based research on traditional forms of grieving and healing. We believed that, if we could understand the traditional forms of healing, we could support a more profound healing process. We had a strong team of four counsellors as part of the project. Margaret and Cynthia were two of the counsellors with whom I worked very closely. Linda was the director of the organization and was one of the initiators of the program.

Margaret is from a small community in northern Ontario of about five hundred people. She has grown children, and worked for more than a decade as the sole mental health counsellor in her community. She was the first to join our project, and stayed with us until the project ended. Margaret was the counsellor who became known for writing excellent clinical reports; the one who would be curious about most everything that was being offered and taught; the one who could bring the details of her personal history to enrich our work. She had lost a son to suicide and understood the grieving and healing process only too well. She shared her own journey of healing and also brought to our attention what might have been helpful to her as she grieved.

Margaret and I often worked together as a clinical team. One specific, very dramatic occasion remains clearly etched in my memory. We were spending a few days in a community of about five hundred people, working with the chief and Band Council, supporting them in dealing with their personal and communal issues of grief, loss, and healing. It had been a difficult day with many pauses and silences, with some of the men speaking out and others clearly moved, but holding back for reasons of their own. Revelations about losses, alcohol problems, childhood fears, and many personal stories were shared that day.

Our team was staying at the nursing station, a comfortable place with staff that we had grown to know. We had a quiet supper and had gone off to sleep. Shortly after midnight, the phone rang with an emergency call. We were told that a young woman in her early twenties had barricaded herself in her house, shotgun in hand. We were told that she was threatening to kill herself or anyone else who might come near her, and that the caller needed our help to talk with her and calm her down. It was not clear whether the young girl was intoxicated.

Margaret and I hurriedly dressed and joined other community members on a small school bus that had arrived to take us all to the other side of the community where the girl's house was located. The ride was completely surreal and otherworldly. In the midst of the anxiety and tragedy of the situation, we drove into the magical night of the northern lights, across shadowy lanes, with trees shimmering. I still remember the brilliance of the sky, lights exploding. All of this was happening simultaneously with our anxious discussions as we developed a strategy to help the young woman.

It was a long night. We called upon the RCMP, but they could not arrive till morning. We had many telephone conversations with the young woman, but were not successful in persuading her to come out. I stood on the other side of the window where she was standing. I then dropped to the ground and crouched low as I remembered that she had a shotgun in her hand, fearful for my own safety. Margaret was constantly present on the sidelines, giving us all ideas on how to proceed, supporting the whole team with her calm and experience.

Later that night, we were able to contact the girl's brother and brought him on the scene. Finally, we had something to bargain with. She was willing to speak with him. Her brother helped us to piece together her story. She had been away from the reserve down south for a few years and had just returned. That very night, she had a serious falling out with her mother and then went into the house, shotgun in hand. It was a blessing that she still felt trusting towards her brother and was able to hear his words of comfort. As a team, we worked with the brother, sharing strategies with him that might help to calm his sister. After several hours of conversation, she was finally willing to put her gun away. She allowed us to enter her house. She was obviously distraught, hair wild, eye-make up running down her face, and very thin. We spoke with her quietly in the house for a while. It was as if her energy was spent and she could not put up any more resistance. We took her to the nursing station where she could sleep. The next morning she was flown out to the hospital a few hundred miles away.

As we were driving back to the nursing station, now about 4 A.M., Margaret looked at me and giggled, saying; "Okay, great expert, now we see what scares you!" She was remembering how I dropped to the ground out of fear when I remembered the girl had a gun. It was a poignant moment, a recognition of how scary and surreal the evening had been, and that here, in the middle of a crisis and in the middle of the night, the roles of expert, professional, counsellor, white woman, native woman, these were all just roles and labels. The reality is that we were all engaged together in a profound moment, and the fact that I was a professional in one particular area of skill could still leave me very vulnerable in other areas of life. I loved being teased like this; it helped me to feel a real connection with Margaret. I was teased for weeks about this, and usually, I enjoyed it!

When I reflect upon the health and mental health issues that face some First Nations women, I am sometimes overcome by a feeling of sadness. There are many problems, with solutions that are not easy, not visible, and certainly, not immediate. Most of us are familiar with the problems of addictions, physical and sexual abuse, depression, and violence that affect First Nations women. We are familiar with the stories of children taken from their homes at young ages to go to residential schools, of what was suffered in residential school in terms of humiliation and abuse, and of the many families that were torn apart by this practice. Many children were taken from homes that would have nourished them and sustained them, and when these children became parents, they had to make a choice to learn to become parents.

I worked with children who were emotionally bereft because their own parents had not been well parented and needed all of their energy and focus to take care of themselves. In these families, it was the children who were sometimes the caretakers, as roles were reversed; what we sometimes call "parentifed children." Sometimes we would have family sessions in which both the parents and the children had to relearn their proper roles.

The goal was to change the dynamics so that the parents were the caretakers, and the children were the recipients of care. The women I have seen in counselling have wanted to mother their children with love. Sometimes it was within their ability to do this, while at other times it eluded them, but they wanted to learn. For many of the women I met, it was the desire to be good parents to their children that became a strong motivation for their own personal healing.

Many of the women, like Margaret, are the keepers of the faith that love can be possible under very difficult circumstances, that hope can be reborn, and that someone can return to light from a very dark and lonely place. The humour and perspective of women like Margaret certainly taught me more deeply about these qualities. The tools that clinical psychology can offer, and there are many useful tools, need to be located in the context of compassion and wisdom for them to be truly useful and to sustain change in another human being. In the literature on spiritual psychology, or transpersonal psychology, the qualities of compassion and presence are being recognized as essential forces within any healing relationship and healing process.

In providing healing, it is necessary to have a clinical diagnosis to inform an appropriate treatment plan. It is essential to know if someone has a personality disorder, schizophrenia, clinical depression, or an anxiety disorder. The tools of psychology are useful, but they need to be joined with true caring and compassion. It is important to believe that the other can in fact heal, even in the face of overwhelming odds. Again, and again, we were shown that when there was a sense of hope and compassion, along with good clinical tools, the client was far more likely to make a good recovery.

These qualities of hope and humour were very much in evidence in a healing circle that we carried out in another community. This particular community, with a population of about eight hundred, had lost several young people to suicide during the previous year. As a community, they were in a deep state of grief so strong, that I literally felt it, like a curtain of sadness, descending as I stepped out of the airplane.

The healing circle was made up of about twenty women who were elders, mothers, and young women. We spoke of what the women had witnessed, and what they were feeling. I spoke about other communities and the efforts they were making to heal and to prevent further suicides, and about the process of grief and healing. The most miraculous aspect of this experience for me is that the healing circle was in Oji-Cree, a language of the northern Ontario First Nations. Everything was translated back and forth, to and from English. While I understood most of the words that were spoken, I certainly missed some of the dialogue. But the spirit of the meeting was impossible to miss: we had created a sacred circle in which women were speaking, thinking, and feeling. The tone was reverent and humorous; the tears were mixed with laughter.

Once again, I was learning more deeply about the wisdom of caring communicated through translation and through body. I felt enriched by the experience. I remember that I was teased about how I liked sitting cross-legged on the floor, yoga-style, which is one of my favourite positions. And this too was an experience of shared connection.

It was from other First Nations women I met that I have learned a great deal about vision and justice. I met Cynthia when she became a counsellor with our program. She was a community organizer, and she continued her work as a teacher of traditional First Nations culture. She had excellent political radar and was able to quickly see through surface nonsense and perceive things in their true light. In her response to me, I found that I was on trial for a while. She eventually decided I might be acceptable.

She brought particular strengths to the project, which I would describe as qualities of justice and political inquiry. When I presented psychological ideas or concepts, I knew that Cynthia might be the first to challenge them. She would want to be shown the real value of some concept or tool, and to really understand its application, before she would see it as useful in our context.

Cynthia also brought a quality of fearlessness to our team. When we went into a new community to introduce the project, she would often be the first one to make contact, to organize how we might proceed in a particular community to help them in their grieving process. Cynthia also led traditional teachings and sweat lodges, and many times brought the beauty and depth of the teachings to our work together. Sometimes we did not agree, and sometimes she did not agree with the management of the program in terms of policy and procedures. On the positive side, we always had an opportunity to discuss matters fully and, generally, were able to come to some amicable agreement about how to proceed. Our project worked in several communities, each one with its own particular needs and cultural style, and we would try to find a unique way to engage each community. We were always inventing the process as we went along, and this aspect of our work was very creative and rewarding.

In thinking about Cynthia and her role in our team, I know I learned more deeply about the value of mental clarity, political savvy, and the importance of earning respect through one's work and value, not through one's professional role. I also enjoyed working with her immensely.

Another woman who had a great impact upon me was Linda, the program director. Linda could be described as fiery, brilliant, vulnerable, and committed. It was Linda, along with the clinical director of the agency, who had developed this project and had had enough faith in me to bring me on board. We had met, Linda, Jonathan (another staff member) and I, over breakfast in a downtown Toronto hotel.

I wanted to learn more about the program, they wanted to learn more about me. I had not worked much in the First Nations community, and I had a pretty fresh doctorate in psychology under my belt. But the chemistry was obviously right, and by the end of our first breakfast together, we agreed to join forces. I am still not certain of the chemistry or the divine plan behind all of this, but within a month, I began my monthly trips to northwestern Ontario.

It was with Linda and Jonathan that we developed our program, our goals, our training materials, and developed the rest of the team. Linda first took me to many of the communities where we would be working, in order to familiarize me with the communities and to introduce me to the chief and council in each area. Linda and I also spoke on a personal level, sharing good stories, dinner, and swimming in clear summer lakes. I remember one memorable night where we went to the church dance on the reserve, with strobe lights ablaze. We also had many meetings with Linda and Jonathan over blueberry pie at a local restaurant in town to debrief our visits and plan for our next trips north into the communities.

Linda herself came from a northern Ontario community that had seen its share of violence, trauma, and loss. She had seen many of the problems that are faced by small northern communities, such as alcoholism, solvent abuse, unemployment, and family problems. Linda's vision and strength served her well in leading the program. She was gifted with stamina and a breadth of scope on how these problems might be solved. We discussed the historical, political, economic, and cultural aspects of these problems and brain stormed about mental health problems that would focus on cultural renewal, traditional values, and supporting the strength of young people. We lamented the deaths that had occurred and were still occurring. And when we were exhausted by our own sadness, we laughed and made jokes with our colleagues about our own and other's little foibles.

I was happy that Linda had hired me, taking a chance on an unknown, white psychologist from the south. When I started this work, little did I realize that I would be working in the north for years to come, as well as in other First Nations communities.

Since my work on that project, I have continued my work in First Nations communities and have continued to meet remarkable women. In my work in Kettle and Stoney Point First Nations, I was called in as part of the emergency team following the death of Dudley George. I stayed on following the crisis and worked closely with one of the women who was working with families in the community. We talked many times of how we could develop programming for children into the community and were successful in implementing some of our ideas. I also worked regularly in the high school and met with the principal to explore how traditional teachings could be incorporated further into the classroom and how I might, in my clinical work, incorporate traditional native myths and stories. When my contract with Kettle Point came to an end, I was gifted with a beautiful feathered, leather dream catcher which now hangs just inside my doorway. It serves as a welcome to all of the guests who enter my home.

I have had the opportunity to work with another visionary woman, Lillian. She brings her knowledge and practice of traditional ways into the setting where she works, and into our conversations. We talk about how we might create a more integrated healing program, which honours both the First Nations traditional ways and values, together with the clinical knowledge of Western psychology. We speak on many levels: philosophical, psychological, cultural, and spiritual, and have tried to create a space that is big enough to contain several traditions. I feel honoured to have shared these conversations with her, and to have brought my knowledge to the clinical setting. My journey with the women of the First Nations continues. I have been the professional psychologist, the student, the colleague, team member, and sometimes friend. I have been in situations that I never dreamed of when I was in graduate school, and have been faced with mental health problems and issues that are far outside the confines of traditional Western psychological knowledge and practice. I have expanded my knowledge, and I have deeply expanded my heart. I feel a deep sense of gratitude for all of these powerful experiences and the many native women who have reinforced my own beliefs that the qualities of compassion, humour, and commitment are central to the fabric of the work of healing. Mental health is a technical term, and it is necessary to expand it and place it within a much larger frame of reference that includes realities like wisdom, connection, healing, and a most radical concept: Love.

Endnotes

1   These names are all pseudonyms for the women, for reasons of confidentiality.

When the Body Attacks: A Black Woman's Fight against Lupus

CHARMAINE CRAWFORD

My mother and I were the best of friends. But nothing had prepared me to take care of her when she became severely ill and disabled in 1999. I was used to her being independent and forthright, not weak and needy. The Black superwoman had lost her cape, and I wished deep down that she would find it and transform herself back into the woman I knew. This is my mother's story, as told through me, in recognition of her courageous fight against lupus.

Eleven years ago, my mother was diagnosed with systemic lupus erythematosus, or simply lupus. Lupus is a debilitating chronic illness that is impeding the life of many women, especially Black women. Lupus is a disease of the immune system that causes damage to the skin (discoid lupus) and/or the joints, nervous system, kidneys, heart, and lungs (systemic lupus). Basically, the body produces anti-bodies that attack healthy cells causing inflammation in connective tissues.

Lupus is fifteen times more likely to occur in women than in men and is twice as likely to affect Black women than White women. Although the cause of this disease is unknown, genetic and environmental factors are attributed to it. This could be a starting point in uncovering why African-Caribbean and African-American women are pre-disposed to this disease. So far, there is no cure for lupus.

Growing up on the Caribbean island of Trinidad, my mother was a sickly young woman who had many fainting spells under the rays of the tropic sun. Upon migrating to Canada in her adult life, she had numerous health problems which doctors could not pinpoint to any one illness or disease, until 1989 when she was diagnosed

265

with lupus. This is a common scenario because this disease tends to mimic the symptoms of other diseases, making diagnosis difficult. This is why lupus is called the disease of one thousand faces. Depending upon the severity of the disease, symptoms may vary to include: skin rashes and lesions, sensitivity to the sun, hair loss, mouth ulcers, inflammation of the joints and/or organs, fatigue, mood swings (agitation and depression), psychosis, and even temporary memory loss

Since my mother's diagnosis, she's had three major flare-ups, with the third being the worst causing long-term debilitation. In January 1998, my mother was down with the flu. After a week or so of not feeling better, she contacted her rheumatologist. My mother knew more was going on with her body than just persistent flu symptoms. She was experiencing joint pains, and rashes were appearing on her skin. After being examined and undergoing a series of blood tests, her specialist told her that her lupus was very active. Put simply, she was out of remission.

Since the disease needed to be treated aggressively, my mother was advised to increase her daily medication (which is a potent anti-inflammatory drug or steroid called *prednisone*). She reluctantly agreed, considering the severe side effects of this drug. This drug, in high dosages over the long-term, contributes to hypertension, diabetes, osteoporosis, weight gain, headaches, agitation, depression, memory loss, and increases susceptibility to infections. My mother was forced into premature menopause at the age of thirty-nine due to drug related side effects. The outcome of using this drug is a zero sum game: you can't survive without it, but your body slowly deteriorates as a result of it.

A month or so later, after being down with the flu, my mother was feeling a little bit better, but she was experiencing swelling and discolouration in her left foot. She went back to her specialist and was immediately hospitalized. She had developed a massive blood clot in her foot that needed to be treated immediately in order to prevent amputation or other severe medical complications. It was later that I found out that it was simply negligence on my mother's rheumatologist's part in failing to prescribe a blood-thinning drug to stabilize the potency of the prescribed anti-inflammatory drug (*prednisone*) which, in high dosages, has the potential to induce blood clots. My mother eventually fired this so-called specialist after she realized he cared little for her well-being.

After spending three weeks in the hospital, one-week bed-bound and the other two going through a series of tests and receiving physiotherapy, my mother got the green light to go home. She left the hospital in her favourite outfit and with a fancy black cane as a walking aid, determined to get her life back on track. I was inspired by her determination and never questioned her ability to bounce back because she always overcame adversity.

My mother was not well enough to return to work so she had to apply for long-term disability to support herself. Her monthly income was reduced. For a working class Black woman, that meant "making do" with a lot less. Having a true warrior's spirit, my mother was set on making the best out of an unfortunate situation. One of her mottos was "Where there is a will there is a way." While at home, she made many lifestyle changes to help improve her health. Since my mother always enjoyed walking, she took short walks to the park, and fruit and vegetable market as a form of exercise. She also modified her nutritional habits and prepared healthy tasty meals that were low in salt and fat. There was also an abundance of fresh fruits and vegetables to snack on. Changing her eating habits was necessary because she had become insulin-dependent as a result of her medication. In order to counter the domino effect of drug-related side effects, my mother met with a licensed nurse and practitioner of homeopathic and naturopathic medicines who prescribed tonics to combat the high level of yeast in her body that was depleting her immunity system. Later, my mother testified that her body felt better. Even her specialist was amazed at her increased strength and vitality.

With so much time on her hands, my mother kept busy to keep from worrying about her condition. She was a master organizer. Put a disastrous situation in her midst, whether it is household clutter or the trials of life, and she would try to fix it or at least put it in order. To pass time, my mother ended up organizing items and rearranging light furniture in her apartment. She spent many hours on the phone counselling her friends on their relationships and chatting about the latest episode of her favourite soap opera. But she eventually grew restless of her new sedentary lifestyle. She was used to being on the move, and coming from a large family, she longed for the company of her family in the US. She visited her sisters in New Jersey and her brother in Florida during the summer of 1998. But it was while she was in Florida that she noticed that her legs were getting weaker, to the point that she could not support her own weight.

By November of 1998, an MRI test confirmed that my mother had dislocated discs in her back which were impeding her mobility. She thought back to a year prior when she'd slipped and fallen on ice during wintertime. After the accident, she was sore for a few days but did not seek medical attention since the pain did not persist. However, with her lupus being active, and experiencing the first signs of osteoporosis, it was a just a matter of time before the effects of her injury surfaced. Her specialist referred her to a surgeon who confirmed that she needed surgery to prevent permanent paralysis. My mother was distraught over this and she thought long and hard before agreeing to have surgery. I, on the other hand, was in shock and downplayed the situation to keep sane.

During the time of diagnosis and subsequent surgery (four months), my mother's condition got worse. Her body was not holding up to all the stress and trauma. She had severe joint pain, but the worst possible thing happened; she developed inflammation in her brain. Her lupus had invaded her brain (which is a minor form of brain disease). My mother lost most of her hair at the back of her head. She became delusional, agitated, paranoid, and had involuntary movements of her head. In turn she cursed and said offensive things to people, both friend and foe. My mother could not sleep at nights and had screaming fits during the day. But, worst of all, some days she did not even recognize me. Basically, my mother thought she was going mad and just wanted to die. While hospitalized, depending on her emotional or psychological state, she was given sleeping pills, anti-psychotic, and/or anti-depressant drugs which often left her in a trancelike state. It was difficult to see my mother so confused and drugged. I felt totally helpless. I could not do anything to stop the demon that was destroying her mentally and physically. By March 1999, my mother was completely bedridden. She could not walk and was incontinent. She developed painful bedsores, which eventually turned into deep wounds due to infection. My mother hated the condition that she was in, but amidst the depression and anger, she was not willing to give in to the disease that was slowly destroying her. She was determined to wage a fierce fight to the end.

From February of 1998 to March 1999, my mother was hospitalized over seven times. I was an emotional wreck, but I held everything within because I needed to be strong for my mother. Our social roles as mother and daughter became reversed, not by choice but out of necessity. At thirty, I was faced with the challenge of mothering my mother. This was not an easy task considering the fact that my mother was a true superwoman who had independence stamped on her chest. I was not used to seeing her helpless, confused, and dependent. I was forced to take charge of her finances and help her make decisions about her medical care. I became her ears, eyes, and voice on all matters with bank managers, doctors, and health care professionals. It was difficult for my mother to relinquish a great deal of her power over to me. I felt, and understood, her terror of losing selfhood when we had disagreements over her personal care and needs.

On my meagre graduate-student income and my mother's disability cheque, I budgeted so that all of my mother's needs were met. As for me, as long I had food, clothing, and shelter nothing else mattered. The rest of my life had come to a standstill. But I soon realized that the task of caring for my mother over the long-term would be impossible due to limited financial resources and inadequate health care services. In the last five years, there has been a massive overhaul toof the Canadian medical system that has contributed to hospital bed shortages, nursing staff cuts, long waits in emergency, and reduced community health care services. My mother became a victim of this restructured system, which disregards the health care needs of disadvantaged sick people.

Upon learning of the severity of my mother's condition, the womenfolk (aunts and cousins) in my family in New Jersey took matters into their own hands to ensure that my mother would get the proper care that she needed. One of my aunts and a cousin pooled together some of their savings so that I would have extra money for any additional medical expenses and general upkeep. Since my mother needed round-the-clock care which I could not provide, and home care would not give, my cousin, who is a health care professional, took three weeks off work (two without pay) to care for her. When my cousin left, my aunt came from Trinidad and spent a month. After she left, another aunt came from New Jersey to be at my mother's side. Cards and phone calls poured in. Relatives came and took occupancy in the hospital when my mother was hospitalized for over a month. She may not have received personal attention from the health care staff, but she sure did from her family. I was totally grateful for this extended family support. But despite all of this kinship love, I knew I eventually had to make a decision about my mother's long-term care.

Before my mother had to undergo surgery, one of my aunts broached the subject of my mother staying in New Jersey for a while where there would be more helping hands to take care of her. My aunt knew that I could not keep up with caring for my mother, and placing her in a nursing home was out of the question. My mother wanted to be with her family. She also felt that things would be a bit easier on me if she visited with them for a while. But there was one major obstacle standing in the way: my mother would not have health care coverage in the US and my family was not rich to hire private physicians. A chronically ill person without health insurance might as well be dead. I was not willing to jeopardize my mother's life regardless of good intensions. On an emotional level, I did not want to be separated from my mother. She was my lifeline, as I was hers.

Never underestimate the power of Black women when they are on a mission. One of my cousins in New Jersey contacted a rheumatologist who was a friend of the family. He agreed to take on my mother as his patient after consulting with her specialist in Canada. We eventually worked out a suitable health care plan with a particular hospital for medical assistance. A month or so after my mother had back surgery, she was transported to New Jersey. She was still very weak and needed to have extensive physiotherapy to regain mobility in her legs. My mother stayed by one of her sisters, who along with her adult children (and other relatives) catered to her personal and health care needs. They faced many challenges taking care of her while she fought to recover, but they held strong out of love and respect. Many family members could not handle seeing my mother weak, depressed, and despondent. The helplessness and fear they displayed told me that they finally understood the seriousness of her condition.

During the last seven months of my mother's life, I visited her monthly and we found comfort in each other's presence. I shared with her what was going on in my life and she listened intently. I bought her treats and small gifts that she cherished. She instructed me on what I needed to do for her regarding her "business" (finances). In retrospect, in many indirect ways, my mother was preparing me for the inevitable. On November 16, 1999, my mother's body succumbed to pneumonia and lupus-related complications while her family kept vigil at her bedside. She was only forty-eight years young.

Talking about Our Health: In Our Hardship We Have to Learn to be Strong

WOMEN'S HEALTH IN WOMEN'S HANDS
ROOFTOP GARDENERS

Women's Health in Women's Hands is an anti-racist, pro-choice, and multilingual community health centre for women located in Toronto, Ontario and funded by the Ministry of Health. The centre has been in existence for ten years and is committed to working for immigrant and refugee women, women with disabilities, young women, and older women. Within these groups we prioritize Black women and women of colour from the Caribbean, Africa, Latin America, and south Asia. In an attempt to address the issue of accessibility to health care, due in part to the cultural, linguistic, racial, gender, age, ability, and class barriers embedded within the health care system, Women's Health in Women's Hands Community Health Centre has created a unique model of service provision. The model is based on the understanding that women's health issues are personal, cultural, social, racial, political, as well as medical. This participatory model focuses on enhancing women's sense of well-being in an environment that allows clients to validate each others' definitions and experiences. We understand that women are experts in their own health care, and our analysis of health care needs are based on conceptualizations of health which encompass and incorporate biological, socio-cultural, psychological, and spiritual dimensions of women's lives. This model locates health within the context of psychological realities. We believe that all of these factors have a direct impact on the state of health and well-being of the individual.

The Wheelchair Accessible Rooftop Garden is a program designed to bring women together to participate in activities that allow them to share their knowledge, not just of plants and growing, but also

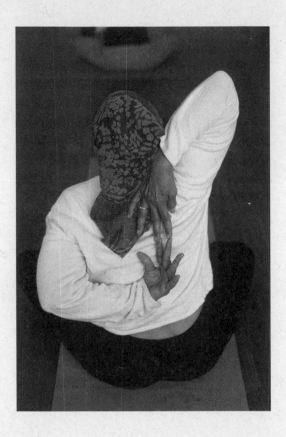

of strategies for maintaining optimum health and happiness. In addition to growing vegetables and herbs to nourish the body, we also grow flowers to nourish the spirit. Workshops on such topics as aromatherapy, relaxation techniques, home remedies, and cultural cooking enhances our sense of well-being. Just being together and forming friendships with each other provides us with the self-support systems we need to carry on.

The following stories have been transcribed (by Kemi Dare) and edited from taped interviews conducted by Linda Cornwell, community health promoter and gardening facilitator at Women's Health in Women's Hands. It has been Linda's very great pleasure and privilege to come to know these women and to learn from them the many strategies and techniques they have developed to remain happy and

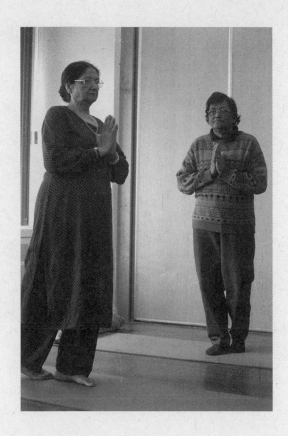

healthy despite the vicissitudes of life. Linda has tried, as faithfully as possible, to preserve the storytellers' own words and their own patterns of speech in order that the stories faithfully reflect the storytellers' realities.

The women in the gardening group were very pleased to meet together to talk about health and to prepare this article that describes the many ways they have learned to care for themselves – body, mind, and soul. So many ways of healing have been scorned, discarded, forgotten, and lost. But now, suddenly at the beginning of the third millennium, people from all cultures are trying to remember and recover all this forgotten knowledge. This is a contribution to the preservation of women's wisdom and a means of sharing the knowledge learned through lifetimes.

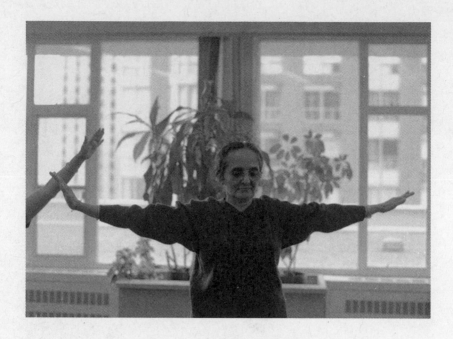

No matter what your condition, think like you are the giant, like you are the best.

SAIDA'S STORY

My name is Saida and I am from Somalia. I came to Canada on August 15, 1991 as a refugee fleeing the civil war. In 1976, I got in a car accident and that left me paralyzed from the waist down, and it also injured my right hand. It was not easy for me to get to Canada because I was in a wheelchair. But my family and the moral support of friends and others that don't even know me stood up and made me possible to come to Canada. My family put a lot of effort and they put all the money they could to put me in a safe place because the civil war was unexpected. I didn't come here for pleasure. I was forced to leave my country.

And it was like this. On November 29, 1990 my father died, and on December 13 my sister was shot in the city, and she died instantly that moment. Her body was brought to us around 11:30 in the morning. And that shocked everybody. And afterwards the whole city was in crisis. I was living in the capital of Somalia, Mogadishu. So, everybody has to leave and go to other places. I went to Kenya and I stayed only twenty-four hours before I passed to Uganda; because at least if you go to Uganda you would be safe. The Kenyans didn't want us because we were having the civil war and everybody was coming. They found out that their economy was going a little bit down, because when you have refugees who don't have homes, they rent from hotels and apartments and whatever they are asking you pay, as far as you can afford, right? So it was too hard for them because you know, their people wouldn't be affording what we could afford.

I stayed in Uganda for almost six months and then I came to Canada as a refugee. The only thing the immigration asked me, when they realized I was paraplegic, I was disabled, they asked me about my diagnosis and that I should go to a neurologist to see my spine and also the urologist. And I was not expecting everything to be perfect for me. I knew that I would have to overcome some difficulties that I would be facing because I left my country and I didn't have any other choice except to be in another country and to look forward. That was all that was possible for me. And what I wanted most was to find a place with accessibility where I could live independently.

When I first came, I lived with my sister in an apartment and then we moved to a house, which was partially accessible because the family who owned it had a disabled child, but it was not fully accessible for a person like me. I had to be with somebody most of the time; my sister or my niece. The toilet was difficult for me so I had to use the bedpan all the time. I didn't want to be a burden to my sister because she has two kids, and she was going to work. My niece was young; my daughter was younger. The thing that helped me move forward was because I was speaking English as I do now, and that helped me a lot. And I found out that Canada is the best place for someone with a disability. I was very lucky. I was able to get a special bed and social assistance to help me survive. When I called Participation Apartments, I was very lucky again; there was an apartment ready.

As soon as I came to Canada, I began going and meeting people and asking them if I can come to volunteer. I met Amina Sharifa who was at York University at that time. She introduced me to many people, and then we decided to make an organization for Somali women. By reaching out, volunteering, helping my community, and getting to know people, I learned many things. Even back home in Somalia I would go to this hospital for paraplegic people with spinal injuries. When I used to go to them, they would say, "How many years you are like this?" because they had only been injured in the last month or so. And I would tell them that no matter what, you have to be happy, you have to live for it. I had everything that a girl of my age could have, you know, my father would provide me with everything, not only me, but all his children and, at the same time, I thought that if I didn't reach what I wanted I would never be happy. But all these ambitions, I don't have any more and still I feel happy. I found out that you can be happy, whatever your condition is.

Before my accident in Somalia, I studied hard. I took two courses at the same time and I learned all about range management; that is the management of the herbs, what the animals would eat. Some parts of Somalia, especially the northern land is very dry. So, we learned about rotational grazing, the watershed management, all this and that. But after my accident, I had to change my life.

I know that you can't buy happiness or you can't just pretend to be happy. Happiness comes from the will of God. And that is what I get from God and I am grateful for that. When I got my accident I said to myself, thank God it was me and not one of my sisters, because I knew I had the strength to survive. Because my sisters, when they have even got a little earache, they need the attention of everybody. What keeps me healthy and happy is my independence, my strength that comes from God and from my father. You cannot imagine all that my father and my family gave me.

You know, sometimes when the weather changes, I have pain in the back of my hips, but still I keep holding my bones. I avoid taking tablets because all tablets have got side effects, even Tylenol. The only thing I will take is like Aspirin, something like that. Sometimes I get headaches and then I try to massage my head and my muscles. Or I will ask somebody to massage me, because I do so many things with my left hand, maybe I overdo the capacity of my strength.

When I was growing up, my father would say, drink at midday a lot of lemon with a little bit of sugar and ice. He would say that it would be a disinfectant for us. And also, if you have got a little bit of cold we used to make ginger. You boil water and you put a little bit of sugar and then take ginger and cinnamon, grind them up and steep it. And if you want to put a little bit of milk, you put milk. Back home, our ginger is very hot because we get the dry, dry, dry roots and grind them. It is so fresh and so hot. If you use the powder, it is not so hot. It has lost its senses; it's hotness, its texture, and flavour. So, I grew up using things like this. Ever since I was so young, my father would give us lemonade every day, and also the castor oil to go to the bathroom every Friday.

Unsi (perfumed oils) is also the Somali culture. It elevates your spirits and your soul. And when you use it and you go amongst the other Somalis, they will smell the perfume when you wave your shawl or scarf. And, ooh, they will give you big compliment, you know. And that makes you feel good, that's what you expect when you use the *unsi*.

I would like to tell women a lot about being healthy and happy because I have experienced a lot of things. If you feel, if you make yourself feel that you are useless, you will always remain useless. But if you tell yourself, I can do everything, then no matter what your condition, you can do. So, no matter what your condition, think like you are the giant, like you are the best. Believe that you can do everything that everybody else can do. And with that, you can go ahead with your healthy life and a live a long, long life.

People maybe will show you rejection and if you let them, they will do it. But if you don't let them, they won't. I remember when I first came back home after my accident with my paralysis, I told my mother and my sisters that neighbours, cousins, and friends are going to come to visit me, because now they know that I came back. Tell them outside the house, before they come to me, not to ask me questions, because I don't want to cry. I don't know how to cry and I don't want to cry. And I don't want that you guys cry, because if you guys cry, I am gonna cry.

One day, this friend of mine came to visit. She was my classmate and we used to go out working with the rural people; the nomads that go from one place to another. We would take our tents and go out into the lands with the nomads. Well, she came to see me and she began crying. And I said, "What are you doing? Don't! And dry your eyes. I don't want you to cry. Didn't they tell you not to do these things to me? Why are you treating me like that? You are my friend; you are my classmate; you are my soul mate. Why are you treating me like that? No matter what has been told to you before you come to my home." After that day she never cried in front of me again. So you don't let people drag you down. And when that happens what are you going to do? You just can't let them put you down,

There is no devil, I believe. There is no devil. When you are weak, you will believe anything. God created this world. And He created us. We are all his children, adults too. So, do you think a father loves one child from the other? No, he loves all his children. Just so, God loves all his children. No matter what!

And if this father has got eight kids, two girls and six boys, he wouldn't say yes, I am proud because I have so many boys. It used to be, you know, " I have more boys so that I have my name go on and on," but that is just uneducated. It was barbarian system I would say, the barbarian system. Men are better? No, we are equal. Because when the man goes to do some work, the woman is taking care of the home and, at the same time, she might be pregnant or she might be breast feeding the child. And there is no job more important than raising the children. So God created this world, and we are his children, and we are equal to him. He created us that we should have respect to each other, through the different religions and different cultures that we have.

Wherever you go in the world there is a culture, and there is also a religion based on that culture. So that the community in Asia or in Africa or in northern Europe or Central America, they have their own ethnic culture. And then they have their religion. Because the

Christians that come from South America or Europe, or the Christians that come from China, they have the same religion, but basically their culture is different. Yes. So is the Muslim and so is the Buddhist and whatever other religion. And I believe that God created us to love each other. And to love ourselves too

And to tell you, when I was back home, I didn't even care about the beauty of nature because it was before my accident. And right after my accident I come to Italy. And I realize the Italians would be saying, "Oh, I would like to go to Africa to see all that culture and all that green and all the animals." That's what they don't have. But when I was young I did not see that. I would want to buy fashionable dresses. You see, so you must treasure all you have.

It's different now I come to Canada. It is the last place that people migrate to and I found out that every people brings a piece of their thing, and that is what they treasure. And then, at the same time, they said okay how can I make what I used to have there. Okay, they introduce other plants from other countries, and they bring here in Canada, and that's what the beauty is about; the diversity is the beauty. And being in a multicultural city like here in Toronto, I mean, it gives you more opportunity to be healthier, to be more aware of what is happening or what is going on around, because you have got so many different communities to learn from; so many different choices.

And the only problem I have as a woman with a disability is with the attendant care, because I have to let people into my apartment and into my life in a close way. I have trouble with one individual, not the others because the others are so good to me. And when the workers talk about other people, other tenants, sometimes if they have to clean somebody, you know, they will say they have difficulty because they have to clean, because she eats such and such. They are even insulted over what they eat. That is not fair. I put in their shoes, I know how I would feel. I know that feces is not a perfume, but they choose this kind of job; you don't have to criticize. Yes, you come for your own choice, nobody, nobody you know persuade you, nobody trick you. You know what you are doing with this job. That is really very bad, what they are doing to us people with disabilities. Anybody can be in our shoes! I can clean myself now, but I can see what is going to happen to me after I can't clean myself. We are human beings, we did not look for these things, and we did not earn to be in this condition. We are the children of God, why do we have to be treated like this. And remember, this is Canada; this is the best for people with disabilities.

And I see many people in my community with that high blood pressure and also sugar diabetes, and I think it's the stress. Dietary changes, the different culture, um, more to that is stress, the first thing. And most of them, they don't know the English language when they come and that cause big stress. And diseases come from emotions too in the first instance. Because people are not the same level of strength. It's like you and me were exposed to a certain disease. I get right away, and you never get. Apart from genetics, isolation causes diseases. A lot of isolation that the person has because inside of you there is something that is bothering you and you can't say loud or you can't share with nobody. I think that is where you get any disease, not only the breast cancer, the blood pressure, the diabetes. You know, it is something that you keep inside, inside loneliness.

Let me tell you my example. When I get my accident, if I will be left alone, if I don't have any hope, I will die soon, many, many years earlier than my lifespan. Thanks God to my father and my sisters and everybody around me. Even my neighbours. Because they know I want to be happy and be elevated. So they elevate me. But if my family will let me down, everybody else will let me down, and I would go down. When you have love and attention, you have your health.

Be strong in your faith and believe.

ALMA'S STORY
I am Alma, but I don't think it matters where I come from. I come from all over the place and I have been living in Canada twelve years now. My illness was my accident first, and three years after my

accident I developed a rare type of glaucoma, which I still have, and I'm still coping with that. And then, in 1989, in October, I developed cataract of my left eye and within six weeks it was removed. So it just developed and then the doctor popped it right out. But in my accident when I fell down some stairs I damaged the optical nerve in my eyes and that was on the thirtieth of July 1988. And ever since I have been visually impaired and I have difficulties to get around. When I got the accident I had my own house, but I got the accident and I couldn't pay my mortgage, so I lost the house. The bank took it back and I lost eighty-one thousand dollars. The bank said they was sending letters, but I can't read the letters because I can't see, and I was in and out of the hospital all the time. So that was my difficult time in my life; I lost my house and I lost my eyesight and I can't do anything about it. I had nobody to stand with me and, up till now, I have to make all my decisions for myself. I am fighting all the time. I had no one to call upon, I didn't know who to phone, I didn't know how to turn, or how to do anything, so I just had to let everything go.

And nobody knows if I have a problem or if I am having a hard time because I always have a smile, and I am always easy. I go here and there and keep busy all the time. I do volunteer work and keep busy and if I don't go, I don't know, I might blow my brain with thinking about problems. I have to be doing all the things I do because it keeps me healthy. And that's my life. If I stay home I might blow my mind. It's true. You see, because the thing is ... I am strong person in a sense, you know and I always say, oh, God is good. In spite of my situation I still pull myself together and say God is good; he will keep me good, in fact, and no matter what. God is helping everybody. Each and every one.

Just this summer I got a test for osteoporosis and the doctor said it didn't look good and I was so frightened that something was really wrong. I was so devastated. But I went to Mount Sinai and I get the bone scan tests and I found out everything is okay. And I feel like a weight come off my shoulder. I feel so released, because it was like a burden, I carry this yoke around my neck. Because before that I kept thinking about it, you know, and I can't comprehend how something else could go wrong with me, you know, I don't know how I will take that. And that is why I keep on going out every day, because if I stay alone, inside, in that apartment, I don't know what will happen.

But even though I talk to everybody, I don't really have close friendship with anybody, because, well, one of my main reasons why I don't keep close friendships, is because I can't take rejection, because I feel like my parents – my biological parents – rejected me. Then my foster parents, they left me because of death, right? Now I am on my own, I can't get over it. I can't. So in my situation, I keep my friendship at a distance. It's not that I don't trust people though, it's just that I keep friendship at a distance and that helps me to keep myself healthy and protected

And as for me, my way of being contented is that I am at peace; I am at peace with myself and with my Creator, and I am at peace with the people around me. I don't have no enemies, I don't get angry, and I don't get anxious, and I don't get aggressive, and I don't envy anybody or lust after anything or anybody. You know people think that lust is when you look at somebody with desire, but lust is a thought. Sometimes, lust could be a thought in your mind about somebody. The thought might be greed, or dislike, or covetousness. All of those things are lust; they are like a thought within. You don't have to say it out. So lust is not only saying things or looking at people in a certain manner. It is a thought as well. I learned that a long, long time ago, and I learned that you must try to keep lustful thoughts away. But contentment means that you have a present personality; you are present with people. You should have no anguish or hate against your neighbours or your friends, and you don't brood all the time. You must not be grumpy all the time. This is contentment; you keep your head on your shoulder; you say hello to everybody.

And in my point of view, everybody is equal, because God created everybody in his image and likeness. So each one of us, regardless of our colour or creed, we are all part of God's creation. We are his image and likeness. That's why he created us the way he sees it's best suited, and he put us in a situation where he sees we would fit. So, these things help me to be content.

You see I write a lot of songs and poems and short stories, and I get my inspiration because of my contentment and peace. I love creation and I love nature and I love birds, and water and sun, rain everything like that. I like people too, but I put people second. I look at nature, and creation, and trees, and plants, and birds, animals, and water. I like all those things. It inspires me a lot. Because, maybe because I think people take me for granted, because I am a person, you know, but these things, I am mad about these things, because I get my inspiration to write about these. I look at a plant, a tree, and I could just start to write something about that tree. I could listen to a bird singing, or I could watch the butterflies you know dancing.... It gives me a lot of inspiration inside and it makes me think a lot. I mostly stay to myself. Not that I'm selfish or anything but I am also a private person and I don't put my dirty laundry out.

I never took any kind of medication. Up to this day, I never take any medication, because I don't have the use for taking medication. But I have to put eye drops in my eye for the glaucoma. I have to do my glaucoma drops. That is my only medication. But if I have a headache or anything concerning my body, I drink water at room temperature. I don't drink cold water. It has to be room temperature. I boil my water, I keep it at room temperature, I drink a glass and I lay down, and the headache goes within half an hour. The headache goes, aches and pains go, and that is it. If you are strong in your faith and believe, a drink of water will help you. Just take a glass, drink it, and lie down to rest. Even when I have a little cramps, I take a glass of water and drink it and I lay down.

I try to stay very calm and collected when I speak. I don't talk static. I am not a static person and I don't like to say all sorts of things, all sorts of nonsense. I say specific things and I get right to the point. And I also think giving keeps you healthy. If I have one dollar, and somebody wants it, I give it to them, and if I have one bread, and somebody wants it, I give it to them. Because I know that God always provides.

Giving love makes you keep a better health.

EDNA'S STORY

My name is Edna. I am seventy years old. Well, I never have any hardship back home, because my parents look after me when I was a child, and after my sisters and brothers leave Jamaica, they look after me, very good. They moved to Canada and England and they help me all through the years. They send money; they send me everything. But I always worked hard, hard in Jamaica. I grew tomatoes and I worked in the field and I sold the tomatoes in the market, but still it's not all easy. You just go on working hard. And then my daughters went to Cayman. And then, from Cayman, one is in Canada here and one is in the States. They look after me very good also. But then my daughter send for me to come to Canada and I came in December 1996, and the condition was very bad, so I went to my daughter in the States. But I came back to Canada and it was very, very hard. Oh, it is too bad to mention it. My son-in-law was bad, bad. He was violent, he threatened to kill; he threatened everything.

And it came down on me like a stick. It came down like a stick. I couldn't eat, I couldn't drink, and I couldn't sleep. Sometimes, when my daughter call me she say, "Come," and she say "You eat the food." And I can't lie, I said yes, at that time, and then I put it in the garbage. And then teatime, I went by the mall and good people giving the money and I buy things of it. But I could not eat in my daughter's house with that bad man there.

But it was good after because I got to know Linda and Valerie, the workers at Women's Health in Women's Hands and they helped me. You help me so much. I was able to get welfare and then my own little apartment and from there the family benefits and, then, from there to my pension, and I want you to put that down in my story. Women's Health in Women's Hands, you are so good. Thank you, thank you.

But thank God I never had any bad diseases. Only one time when I went to the doctor to get some pills and he say the cholesterol is high. I went back for tests three times and they don't call me. So, that means to say that it is okay. I don't have the pressure, I don't have the sugar, and my bones are good. And I thank God who is helping everybody, each and every one; yes.

To stay healthy you have to have faith. But you have to help yourself and look after the body too. I think having a right diet, having good exercise and contentment – contentment is one thing to keep healthy, 'cause if you are not contented, no matter what you eat and what exercise you take, it's not going to work. You have to live the good way, with good people, and don't mess around with them bad people. You try to live the right and proper way, how you ought to live.

You see anything that a person eating that is not right, you can say that this not food for them to eat. Eat so and so, and eat so and so, and try to keep healthy. I think that is the best. And then you are contented if you have good health. You don't quarrel, messing with people that get you messed up because then you have to have those burden, and you carrying too much burden from other people. You can't keep up with it that way. And if you feel like you discouraged, you don't want to eat or drink, sometimes you feel like you don't want anything, but yet, by singing or reading or praying, you know, you can just get by. You pray to get back to yourself, and you get back to yourself. If you're with miserable people you can't keep with them, you just cannot.

And you can't do bad to other people and keep a good health, because if I do anything bad to you now and I go home, it rests on me and that gives me bad health. Because I have it on me; I can't sleep, I can't eat, I can't drink. So it, it burdens you so much that you can't have a good health in that way. And we have to love one another to have a good health. You don't hate, you don't try to hate no one. If anyone want to hate you, fine, you can't change that, but you don't try to hate them back.

And when I see a friend crying now, I just feel for her and it can affect my health right away. So, when you see people cheerful it is better for you, because sometimes people respond and discourage you and you, the healthy person, can get that bad energy. You know, it's like a transition of the energy. But you can also give them your good energy. Yes, you can send down your good energy to help other people. And giving love makes you keep a better health. God don't taught men to sin.

And eating good things make you keep a good health. I was talking to a lady the other day and she say, "Are you a senior?" I said "yes," and she said, "No you are not a senior." I said I am. She said, "How old are you?" I said I am seventy. She said, "No, you are fifty. You can't be that, you don't have the wrinkles; you don't have this or that. What you eat? Write down the things that you eat and give me. Give me the recipe, the things that you eat." You see, so when you eat and drink the right thing, you will keep good health. And good health is the best

When I young, I worked hard, I worked hard, but I eat the right thing. Like all those cow foot, cow tail, cook it down to jelly and bottle it up. Then you are ready to go eat-drink. And you take the cow foot and you make soup and you drink it down good. And this cracked corn, this cracked corn is a wonderful thing. It is healthy for your body. It keeps you healthy

And then, there are some of the things what I use back home; like I can get this black mint, all the Trinis get it.... And what I use for tonic back home, I get it here and I use all these same things. Especially I use the aloe vera; I boil it and drink it and it cleans out the body. It helps the blood and it purges you; that means to say, if you have cold in your body, it purges. All like in this country now, where you have to go through cold weather for so long. And you can boil that thing and drink it or, if you want to, scrape it and mix it. But when you boil it and mix, it is better, and then you have this bowel movement. You don't feel that itching in your bones again.

And I drink a lot of sour seed. Sour seed now it cleans your blood and it purifies it. I even have seeds at home here. I don't know if they will grow. But I buy it at the West Indian store and then you have the liquor and the seeds. I take out the seed and dry it. So I don't know if they will grow, but when the spring is out I am going to sow them out and maybe it will grow. Is the thing grow long and climb up, climb up. Some people call it bitter lemon and always the men in Jamaica, when they going to the farm and working and know that they going to get tired, they get the sour seed, and boil it and drink it to help them stay strong. And also I use the thing you call eucalyptus. The tree grows up tall. It's good for colds.

So there is lots of different herbs back home, and when I see them here I get them. There are many things that I know back home, when I go in the store and I see all these bushes and so, sometimes the grocery stores sell it, sometimes the Chinese stores. Even this basil. We call it wild basil. We boil it for tea and we use it for baths too. But even the medicine that the doctor can give to you I don't know, but I pray over it. If I get medicine from a doctor, I pray over it before I take it. I ask the Lord to be help with my body. That's what I do. I pray over the medicine and ask God, let it be available to my body.

You know what will keep you healthy again? Get up early and go and have some morning walk. Get the morning breeze. You don't lay in bed till seven, eight, nine o'clock when the sun raise. In Jamaica, you get up before the sun raise and you go out, and all in the mornings now you have banana leaves. You take the dew from them to wash your face. And even here, now, in the winter, you still come up that action and exercise. Walk up and down in the passage, go down in the lobby or come up the passage. Hold on the railing and exercise and you kick your foot up. And then you bend on down and try to catch your toe and come up back seven times. Good exercise. But you have to keep doing everyday or your body stiffens.

But the minute I feel like I am down, I get on the phone and I call a friend and I talk, and the person talk to me. And yet you may not tell that person that me down. But we talking and we talking and afterwards, oh, everything bad is gone. Talking to people when you really in that bad position is psychological help because you get out of your own focus. There is somebody. You don't say well, this happen to me, but by talking your days are put right. And that just feel good, you see you don't have that trouble on your mind any more.

The other day I was sitting down, waiting for a bus. And a bird just come down and I say my God what is this. And I say Jehovah, I am going to read and I pick up the Bible and John 14 "Let not your heart be troubled." After that I sing a chorus. After that I feel, oh, I feel like I am a baby here. You know. Send the tears away and brighten up the day.

And I like to help people around me. I always say, if there is anything, I can help you, I won't say no. Because I am here to help anyone with whatever I can do for them. I am here, and while I am I can reach to you. That is the way. The help is there; the love is there. Yes, and giving. That is what I tell people and I tell my children. I write my sister and them in England and I tell them the same thing. I say you know why God blessed me so much in foreign country? With good that I do back for you. If I went out and I saw a blind person stopped across the road, I turn back and I try to help him. And if you thief a blind, it better you dead. It come on you like if you hurt a little baby. And that is what I tell my children then. I say the good God will always provide for me. But if you thief a blind, it better you dead. It come in like if your hurt a little baby. You better have me say, hand round your neck. And that is what I tell my children then. I say the good God will always provide for me. And if it is the last cent I have and you beg me, I give you. And by the time I reach home, there so, I get more than the cent.

So good, good food, good faith, good friends, good life, good exercise, all of these things are important. And the more is when we have love with us too.

If you don't have a peaceful heart, you won't have a peaceful house.

MYRTLE'S STORY
I am Myrtle. I had seven babies in Jamaica, and all those babies I had alone in my home and I did not go to the doctor or the clinic except for the last one. All those children, I grew them up by myself. And my life was good in Jamaica, but I always worked hard. I never had no sickness, no trouble. Well, little problems here and there, but no big trouble. Sometimes, a little pain but I would keep on working. And then I came to Canada in December 1991. My daughter, that

is my first daughter brought me here, but since the very beginning, she does not help me at all. I was fifty-eight years old and I had to work, so I got jobs to do babysitting, and look after the children and the homes. I really think it is hard. I know it was for me to be in the new country. Growing up, I among so many people, I have so much friends, you know. And coming here and having no one. Because I have to say, I had no one in Canada. Different country, so much different, so much changes. My children, I can't depend on them you know. But I tried to cultivate steps.

But then, when I get older and I cannot work in the people's houses any more, I did not know what to do. Things wasn't working so, but I keep to myself and the little I have I tried to look after myself. But I had no income and I didn't know how I could pay my rent. But, good thing, I met Ms. Hall who worked for the housing company. And she was talking to the other tenants and after she finish her lecture I went to her and I told her I would like to talk to her. And she put me on to Women's Health in Women's Hands and since then I got my family benefits. But the bad things I try to put them backwards, you know, I don't put them in front. Because if the problems are always put in front, they will get at my nerves. So that's my greatest health, within myself, you understand? I learn myself to be strong. In our hardship we have to learn to be strong.

You know, there is no partiality in disease. Whether you are good or bad, you get disease. Sometimes it is not for any particular type of people. Disease is not meant to be for one class or one particular type of people. Anybody can get any type of disease. It depends. Sometimes, our immune system is low and we have low resistance. And because of the low resistance, any germ in the air, you can catch. But if you have a strong immune system, you can resist. And that is why you must try and keep your body strong. Take care of your body because it is like a temple. I have brought this book and, if you want, you can have a look at it. These are things that I believe in. It is Godly advice. It's called *Science and Health with Key to the Scriptures* and it is Christian Science, which was founded by a woman, Mary Baker Eddy, and she wrote this book. "Ye shall know the truth and the truth shall make you free."

My doctor used to belittle this and she didn't believe in it, but I find is such a nice book to read and it gives me peace. You know, you don't have to be of that religion to read their books, because no religion tell you to do anything bad. Every religion is a path to God.

That is what they preach and study in church. That is why I said to you, everything is coming out more, because in the end, knowledge will increase. What we never use to bring out, all this is coming now, and it works.

But you know, my main problem now is that I can't understand my doctor, because what I go to him for, he is giving me something else. So, I just, you know, I wouldn't say he wouldn't help but I don't really put that much confidence in him, and if you don't put confidence in him he's no help. Well, it is very hard for me because I go to the doctor and then I find I am getting lower and getting sicker. Would you put confidence in a person who you go to him and instead of you get better you get worse? I don't think that is reasonable. He sent me for all these tests and they worry my mind so, and then he said to me there is nothing wrong with me apart from what I told you, the blood pressure and the cholesterol. Even after all the tests he doesn't see anything; no diabetes, no cancer, no heart or this, that, or the other. Well, maybe I would say I have confidence in him, but taking those tablets, seven tablets a day, I don't want to take all those medicine. Like he give me the hormones and then my period come and come. I don't have this since I was fifty and I don't want to have this now at this age. It's not right. And all these tests, that is what I am here suffering from, because it worry me and it weaken me so much when I put my mind on it, and I do not want it anymore. So I stopped taking the tablets and I don't have any cold anymore, I don't have any chest pain any more.

But still, I try to live the good life and keep myself so. I drink the herb teas and I always boil the water and drink hot things only. And I don't complain and try to bring myself low. If I have the little pain, I keep going. All my life I keep going. I have the seven babies and I look after myself. You see I try my own way. As I said, I didn't grow up on doctors and medicine. In my days, there were no doctors.

But I know it is hard for your body, going to a different country, and sometimes I feel to go back home. That's it. This country is hot and then cold. And you know, it is different, all is different; the air, the food, everything. But still the body is there. The same body, the same blood, the same everything.

When I was back home, we used the real Indian food. And we used quinine, Aspirin. And here, when I was feeling the chilly knees and go to the pharmacy to sell me the quinine, they say I will have to get prescription. So, I didn't get it because I know my doctor. I told him about it and he didn't say whether it is a fever or what, even when I suggested. The doctor is not God. He cannot relieve everything.

And what we do back home, we don't have everything on ice. We eat hot food and drink hot teas. And back home you dig your food; you get it fresh. Here now, you buy anything in the store, from the year of one, and you still buying it. But what I said, like we back home, we know what we use for our health. I come here and I buy it. Those things we take them from back home and we take them here to stay healthy. We take the tonic and the iron. The most thing for your body is the iron.

Back home when we had a baby the nurses and midwives looked after you. They were women in the village and they come in like nurse, but they deal with bush, they are bush wife, and they know the herbs. And they bath you after you have the baby. And then after you have baby, you have to stay in your room nine days before you come out and do work. But nowadays, woman have baby today and by tomorrow she's on the street. Back then, after you have the baby you have to bound your belly, you have to wear your particular clothes for how much months before you can take it off, because you can take a cold in your womb. After you have a baby, every joint in you is like this. Every joint, and that's how you take a cold. Because every joint, cold. So, you must keep it all warm.

And that is why we are so healthy now that we are older. Yes, because we try to keep our life. You have to really keep your life. You have to really keep your body in such a way that it can be healthy. If the doctor tells me don't eat these types of food, I want to be healthy so I do not eat it. I like to eat good food and drink teas made from herbs. And for the sweetness, I don't eat the cakes and things; I mostly like bananas, grapes, and fruits because the sweetness is in them.

But maybe these days the young people now, back at home, change over and do not do things like we used to do. Maybe nowadays they think that a pill will cure everything. And you know it can't.

I'll tell you some things that are good for you. You take this rum, proof rum. Cut up some ginger and peel it and put it in there. Or put green pimento in there. And if you can get this thing, the good chilli pepper, put it in there. And you use it when you coming out of the cold or after your shower. You take it and you rub it on your body, on your knees, or wherever you want. And you can drink it too. Just a little, maybe a teaspoon, or a tablespoon. But you take it like medicine; too much drink is not wise.

And back home now, we take the leaf of life; you put it in a glass of water and you drink it and it is a good medicine for healing of the body. When we go healing, they give it to us to drink. Clear pretty water with a leaf of life in it. And then after you drink the water, you take the leaf of life and you suck out the juice. It is good for cold too.

But sometimes your belief has a lot to do with you and your health, what you believe no matter what the doctors say. Sometimes we are pressured, we have the pain, or sometimes we wake up so cranky. And then, I don't take anything. I start over, get the fresh air, drink the warm tea, keep the peaceful feeling, and then I feel good. Peaceful mind is everything, you know.

Even in the hard, hard times, at least the thing we got is we are strong and we try to bear it, and it goes away. If it is a thing that the doctor have to work on you, well, he will try to do his best, but you have to be strong and do the right things, live the right way. When the things are good with us, it helps us, in our body, in our head, in everything. It helps us to know our own people. And to know how to be good to people. Your approach has a lot to do with you. And this approach come from the heart. If you don't have a peaceful heart, you won't have a peaceful house.

I don't go running to other people with every little problem. I keep my feelings close to me until its low down a little and I don't feel it so strong. Then I talk over it, it don't rise a lot. You know sometimes things get you angry and if you talk right away you just angry, angry. It's better to let your feelings low down.

I do believe it is hard for young people today though because everything open up to them. These children now, they know everything and they are seeing too much things, especially in this foreign country. We don't have it back home, all these things you see on TV. All these sex and then these other things, we never see it on TV when we back home. And now when we come here and I see some things on TV, I say oh my God, what is this, too much. And that is why the kids them spoil so much. And them are bringing up children; don't you see babes having babes? Babies having babies now. It's fulfillment of scripture. God has said that when his time is near, babes will be having babes. And it is pure babes having babes now. They should be in school, but they having babies. You never get away from God's law. That is one thing we never can do. Can we imagine these things from when we are little children?

Some Simple Cures from Our Gardening Group

(These home recipes are not intended to replace your doctor's advice. Please check any prolonged or unusual condition with your doctor.)

SORE EYES

Place a thin slice of cucumber on each of your closed eyes. Lie down and relax for twenty minutes or so. This is a really simple way to relieve and revitalize burning and stinging eyes. Cold tea bags are also very soothing. Cold chamomile tea bags calm irritation and allergic reactions.

SOOTHING TALCUM POWDER

These are very good powders for hot days. Talc itself is a mineral that is often irritating and cuts into the skin. Recent scientific studies report that it can be very harmful to the body. Cornstarch and baking soda do not harm the body, and are very useful in baby care.

Grind together one tablespoon of cornstarch, one teaspoon of baking soda, and one teaspoon of finely powdered herb.

Lavender talc is a beautiful scent and is good for the body.

Thyme is good for the feet. For athlete's foot, rub between the toes with lemon peel, releasing the oil, and then dust with thyme talc.

For feet that become overhot and tired, parsley talc is soothing.

MUSTARD FOOT BATH

If your feet become hot and flat after a long walk, or if they are so cold that it seems to eat into the bone, a foot bath can relieve and revitalize the whole body.

Mix together two teaspoons of ground mustard with ten cups of hot water. Soak the feet in this mixture for twenty minutes. Close your eyes and allow the warmth to spread through your body. Dry well and keep your feet warm afterwards.

HAND BATH

Herbalists have examined the efficiency of hand and foot baths and advocate them as a major therapeutic strategy. Use any herb for a bath.

Soak the hands (or any limb) for twenty minutes. The whole body relaxes while the herb is absorbed; simple, beautiful, and efficient.

SAGE AND VINEGAR POULTICE FOR SWELLING AND BRUISING

1. Bruise whole fresh sage leaves by flattening them with a rolling pin. Try not to break or tear them.
2. Put the leaves in a pan and just cover with white vinegar. Simmer over very low heat for five minutes. The vinegar should not boil but it should steam so that the leaves will soften and blanch.
3. After five minutes, take out the leaves and lay them on a cloth. Work quickly and carefully as the leaves are very hot. Fold the cloth into a package that will just cover the affected area.

Apply as hot as you can stand it and cover with towels to retain the heat. Leave on for an hour or so until the swelling has subsided.

VINEGAR AND BROWN PAPER POULTICE
This is a very old-fashioned remedy for swelling and bruising.

Put five or six sheets of strong brown paper in a saucepan and cover with (any kind of) vinegar. You can add a bit of sage. Put the lid on and simmer over very low heat for a few minutes until the paper is softened. Do not let the paper break or disintegrate.

Take paper out and wrap it around the affected area in overlapping layers. Use it as hot as possible and build up several layers. Cover with plastic wrap and bandage. Leave on for four hours. Vinegar poultices feel very supportive and strengthening. Reapply twice a day until the swelling and bruising have subsided.

FIGS
Figs are nutritious and easy to digest, but they are probably best known for their gentle laxative action. Adding a few chopped figs to your breakfast cereal is a good way to increase the fibre in your diet and to ensure regularity. The long-term treatment for constipation

is, of course, to eat more dietary fibre, such as fruit, green vegetables, and wholegrain cereals. Syrup of figs is a popular standby for occasional use.

Figs have also been used for treating skin diseases for many centuries. Twenty-seven hundred years ago, the prophet Isaiah advised King Hezekiah to treat his boils with mashed figs. The milky white juice that comes from the stalks of fig leaves is said to be a cure for warts. Ointments and creams made from fresh fig leaves are healing and cooling for itchy skin problems.

SYRUP OF FIGS
8 Dried figs
1 Cup of water
1 Cup of molasses or brown sugar
Juice of two Lemons
1 Teaspoon of ground ginger

Slice figs thinly and simmer in water until soft; about twenty minutes. Pour off the liquid and set figs aside. Make liquid back up to the original amount with fresh water, add molasses and heat gently, stirring all the time until the sugar is dissolved. Add lemon juice, ginger, and figs and blend in a blender or food processor. Pour into sterilized jar, label, and store in a cool place. It will keep well. Dose: for a child, one to two dessertspoons daily; for an adult, three to four dessertspoons daily.

GEL ALOE
Wash two large leaves of aloe.
Slice and scrape out the flesh into a large basin, then blend and throw it into a pan. Mix in one pint of stout. Bottle the mixture in a clean jar and refrigerate.
Dose: one tablespoon daily.

Alternative #1 Boil scraped aloes in two quarts of water. Boil down to one quart. Strain and set aside to cool. Bottle and store in refrigerator. Drink like water with no sugar added.
Dose: One wine glass full per day.

Alternative #2   Scrape out aloes as above and mix with a little condensed milk. Prepare as much as you are going to drink this way and store remainder in the refrigerator. Prepare as needed by mixing stored aloe with milk.

FRUIT VINEGAR
Sterilize bottle.
Cover fruit or berries with vinegar and leave to stand for two weeks. Strain and bottle in sterilized jar.
To use: one teaspoon to a cup of water or to taste. Fruit vinegar is sharpening and cleansing first thing in the morning – a Wake-up tonic for the whole body. In winter, you can use fruit vinegar to ease coughs and colds, to cut phlegm, and to soothe fevers.
Iced fruit vinegar is cooling and soothing on a hot summer day.
It is best to make fruit vinegar in the summer when soft fruits and berries are plentiful. This is an easy way to preserve their minerals and vitamins for use in the cold, dark winter, when fresh fruit is very expensive.

HERB VINEGAR
Herb vinegars can be made the same way as fruit vinegars. Use one ounce of dried herbs or two ounces of fresh herbs in two and a half cups of vinegar.
   A vinegar hair rinse keeps the hair scalp healthy and hair conditioned. Dilute one tablespoon of herbal vinegar in one cup of water. Rub thoroughly into the scalp. Leave for five minutes and then rinse off. Use sage to darken hair or chamomile to lighten it. Parsley helps cure dandruff, and rosemary is good for dry, thin or falling hair.

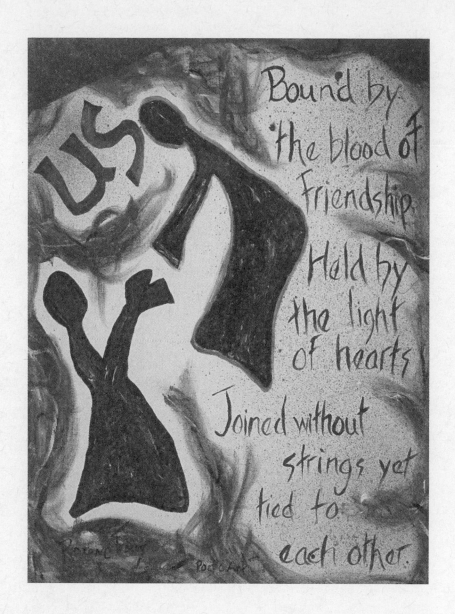

Notes on Contributors

BYLLYE AVERY was heralded as the "Guardian of Public Health" by the magazine *American Health*. It is an apt description for the visionary behind the Avery Institute who also co-founded the Black Women's Health Project some twenty years ago, as well as the Gainesville Women's Health Center and Birthplace in Gainesville, Florida. She is currently a Clinical Professor in the Heilbrunn Department of Population and Family Health at the Mailman School of Public Health at Columbia, University.

Ms. Avery is also a recipient of the Dorothy L. Height Lifetime Achievement Award and the President's Citation of the American Public Health Association, and a leadership award from the University of Florida's School of Medicine. In 2003, she received the Lifetime Television Trailblazer Award. What grew out of Ms. Avery's rich experience at Harvard was the plan for the Institute, an organization that would promote community approaches and support community and scholar activists in an atmosphere that defines health issues from the community's perspective, and targets social justice and equity issues in healthcare, particularly for women of colour. The Avery Institute for Social Change emerged from her two-year stay as a Visiting Fellow at The Harvard School of Public Health's Department of Health and Social Behavior after she was awarded the MacArthur Foundation Fellowship for Social Contribution. This recognition honoured Ms. Avery's years of work developing programs to improve the health and self-esteem of black women.

DR. WANDA THOMAS BERNARD is a life-long African-Nova Scotian. She has a BA from Mount St. Vincent University, an MSW from Dalhousie, and a PhD from the University of Sheffield (England). A founding member of the Association of Black Social Workers, Wanda is an Associate Professor and Director at the Maritime School of Social Work, Dalhousie University. She has done extensive research work with Black Men and is currently conducting research on the impact of racism and violence on the health and well-being of African-Canadian men, their families, and communities in Halifax, Toronto, and Calgary. Previous research topics have explored topics such as Africentric perspectives in social work, race relations in the education sector in Nova Scotia, and issues of addiction and health care services with African-Nova Scotian women.

DR. ANA BODNAR is a clinical psychologist who has been working in the First Nations community since 1992. She is based in Toronto, where she has worked as an educator, consultant, and psychotherapist. She has taught seminars in many First Nations agencies, as well as teaching in the areas of creativity and spiritual psychology for the University of Toronto, the YWCA, the Centre for Addiction and Mental Health, Sheena's Place, Canadian College of Naturopathic Medicine, Leading Edge Seminars, and others. She acts as a consulting psychologist to the Aboriginal Services Program at the Centre for Addiction and Mental Health. She also sings, paints, and does sculpture.

SHIRLEY BROZZO is Keweenaw Bay Anishnaabe from Marquette, Michigan. She is currently employed at Northern Michigan University, where she coordinates a retention program for all students of colour on campus. She is also an adjunct instructor with the Native American Studies Department. Shirley has earned a BS in Business Administration and an MA in English writing, both at NMU. She has had over twenty-five poems and short stories published.

My name is NORA BURRELL; I was born in Jamaica and emigrated to Canada. I have lived in Canada for more than twenty years. I am the mother of four children. I look to God for strength and comfort in all things.

BISHAKHA CHOWDHURY: The two poems which I submitted for this book are about a very sorrowful and painful part of my life, and it has taken me some time to feel that I can share them with a wider circle, past my family and close friends. The first is about feeling spiritually bereft and of searching for a way to return to the sense of spiritual fullness and wellness. I wrote this poem on the due-date of my baby girl, whom I had lost at twenty-one weeks of pregnancy. The second is written in the style of a *haiku* and is about finding the beginnings of the healing process actually contained in the depths and darkness of sorrow and pain. I have been fortunate to have a beautiful child since this loss and his presence in my life, along with that of my first child, is of immense importance as I continue to journey along the road of healing.

LINDA CORNWELL is a Community Health Promoter at Women's Health in Women's Hands. She works primarily with older women and with women disabilities from ethno-racial communities by delivering programs designed to promote healthy living and also by providing individual advocacy support to ensure that all women receive their just entitlements. She has prepared and presented briefs and papers on a variety of issues impacting on the health of immigrant/refugee women, including responses to the House of Commons Standing Committee on Citizenship and Immigration Issues and the House of Commons Standing Committee on Justice and Legal Affairs on the legal implications of including Female Genital Mutilation in the Criminal Code. She has also written and presented papers on elder abuse in ethno-racial communities; culture, race and disability; the impact of globalization on people with disabilities, and female genital mutilation eradication strategies. Linda is a board member of Ethno Racial People with Disabilities Coalition of Ontario, a member of the National Action Committee on the Status of Women Southern Ontario Steering Committee, and a member of various committees working for social justice.

CHARMAINE CRAWFORD is a graduate student in Women's Studies at York University, Toronto. She is committed to doing further research on black women and Lupus.

KAREN FLYNN is the director of the Women's Studies Program at St. Cloud State University. She has published in the area of violence against Caribbean women, Black women and poverty, and Caribbean immigrant nurses. Her research interests include women and work, racism, feminism, and post-colonial theory. Karen also writes a regular column for the community publication Share.

RANDA MINA HAMMADIEH is of Syrian origin, and she currently resides in Miami with her Cuban husband Louis Bensa, where she is the executive vice-president for Glorious Destiny Records. She would like to dedicate her work firstly to John Menga (r.i.p.) of Toronto who was brutally murdered by the Toronto Police force getting into his car in broad daylight. She would also like to dedicate this to Louima Abner, Dudley Laws, Otto Vas, and anyone else who has ever been a victim of police brutality and aggression.

(GRISSELDA) SOPHIE HARDING is a student and employee at York University, Toronto. Her writing is an expression of her desire to change the world and help make life better for herself and others. She believes that love, giving, and caring for people is the key to happiness and success. Her goal is to continue to grow spiritually, emotionally, and mentally, always learning as she travels on the journey of life. Sophie's first anthology is entitled: *Our Words/Our Revolutions Di/Verse Voices of Black Women/First Nations Women and Women of Colour in Canada* (Inanna Publications and Education Inc., 2000). Some of Sophie's work has been used in projects such as the Teen Violence Prevention Initiatives with Women's Habitat; this project produced an interactive CD-ROM and video that are used in schools to educate students about dating violence. Her work is also featured in the *Women, Violence, and Adult Education Project (World Education) Source Book*, which is aimed at examining the effect of violence in terms of learning and education for women. Her mother and her husband continue to be her backbone and a constant supply of daily inspiration.

CIAJDIANN HARRIS is a journalist, poet, and freelance writer residing in northeast Ohio. A paralegal and former state law enforcement officer, Ciaj currently works part-time as a staff writer for the *Chronicle-Telegram* newspaper in Elyria, Ohio, and part-time as a substitute teacher in the Lorain Public school system. She recently completed work on a collection of poetry, short stories, essays, and life lessons entitled *I Count It All Joy*. One of her works appeared in the 2001 United Nations anthology *Dialogue among Civilizations through Poetry*. She also will be featured in the upcoming anthology I Finally Woke Up and Put on My Crown. Ciaj realized her "Dream Deferred" when she was admitted to law school at Cleveland State University, Cleveland-Marshall College of Law for 2004.

LAYLA HASSAN is a childhood cancer survivor and mother of a fabulous two year old. She attends the University of Western Ontario. She plans to attend teacher's college (yet is still trying to figure out how an amputee does such things). She is a queer, one-legged (hemi-pelvectomy), bi-racial Arab-Canadian searching for that perfect leg. She lost her leg at the age of nine and had a second surgery at eleven. Recently fitted with a prosthetic leg, she is learning to walk yet again. Among other subjects, she writes about such experiences as being a cancer survivor, a woman with a disability, a mother, queer, married, bi-racial, passing as white, life in between and being mistaken for everything she is not.

TROY HUNTER is a photographer, freelance journalist, multimedia artist, and historian. He is a member of the Ktunaxa Nation of southeast British Columbia. Hunter has collected oral histories along with accompanying portraiture. Hunter is known for a collection of Ktunaxa oral histories published in 1999 by the Ktunaxa Independent School Society but more so for his regular contributions to British Columbia's Aboriginal newspaper *Raven's Eye*. He is a self-taught photographer whose experiences began when a Ktunaxa elder gave him an antique roll film camera in the mid-1970s. Hunter is the recipient of various awards for his documentary art.

ROLANDA CHAVETT KANE is a Nova Scotia-born universal articulate Black womanist poet and mother of one (Suella Madeline Kane). She is currently involved in several local artists organizations and continues to have many links with the African continent through her work. She views her poetry as the yolk in the power and centre of her voice.

ROSAMOND S. KING is a poet, scholar, and paper artist. The poems published here are from the Endo Poems, which detail the experience of living with endometriosis. King's creative work has appeared in a number of journals, including *Xcp: Cross-Cultural Poetics*, *The Caribbean Writer*, *Another Chicago Magazine*, and *Poet Lore*, as well as in anthologies such as *Beyond the Frontier: African-American Poetry for the Twenty-First Century*. King serves as Business Director of Witness Tree Literary Arts Education, Inc., and proprietor and Factotum of Eating Artist Services.

Metis writer, HEATHER SIMENEY MACLEOD's first book of poems, *My Flesh the Sound of Rain*, was published in 1998 by Coteau Books and was nominated for the First Nations Publishing prize that year. A chapbook, *Shapes of Orion*, published with Smoking Lung Press was released in 2000. Two of her plays have received honourable mentions from, the journal, *Aboriginal Voices* and from the Native Playwrights Contest held in Alaska. She has a second poetry collection, *North Woods* (a collaboration with Coral Hull) forthcoming with Rattapallax Press. Heather's third poetry book will be released with Turnstone Books in April 2004. Her work has been published widely in Canada as well as in reviews and journals in the United States, the United Kingdom, Ireland, Australia, Israel, and New Zealand. Heather lives in the interior of British Columbia and is at work on a novel.

MARISA MAHARAJ has been writing since she was young. She dabbles lightly in the quest to get published and for the most part leads a simple everyday existence. A voracious reader, she also enjoys physical activity, good conversation, and spending time with interesting people. She currently resides in Mississauga and works in Kitchener.

KRISTINE MAITLAND is an interdisciplinary private scholar, dancer, dance instructor, writer, and social critic. She maintains a black history website at www.kmaitland.ca and has been previously published in *The Toronto Star, Mix Magazine, Fabula, Moxie Magazine, at the crossroads*, and *Trade!* magazine. She has also appeared in *Strange Sisters, Mayworks, TalkTV*, and CKLN. Ms. Maitland dedicates her article to her mother, Miss Vivienne.

NOTISHA MASSAQUOI is currently the Program Manager for Women's Health in Women's Hands Community Health Centre. She is also a PhD student at the Ontario Institute for Studies in Education/University of Toronto. She has a commitment to the healthcare needs of immigrant and refugee women and in particular is involved in community development, community-based research, and policy development as it applies to the healthcare needs of Black women and women of colour.

NAOMI NORTH is a mixed race, comin' from poverty, feminist, femme dyke activist currently living on the coast of British Columbia. She quietly writes away despair bred through a keen life-long awareness of injustice. As a new mom, she is awed by the depth of love, compassion and hope inspired by pregnancy, the birthing and witness of new life.

SIMA QADEER completed her undergraduate degree in political science and sociology at the University of Toronto where she discovered her passion for social justice and civic activism. Her favourite pastime is travelling. Currently her travels are on hold while she completes her Masters in Public Policy and Administration.

TALATA REEVES has worked in the substance abuse, HIV, and criminal justice fields since 1991. She worked in alternatives to incarceration programs and in the majority of substance-use treatment approaches and settings. She is currently the Director of Women and Family Services at Gay Men's Health Crisis in New York City. Ms. Reeves has a master's degree in Divinity.

CARLA R. RIBEIRO's academic background includes undergraduate and postgraduate degrees in Psychology and Women's Studies from York University in Toronto. She has worked as a counsellor and has served on boards of non-profit agencies that provide services to women and children. The axis of all of Carla's work has been the belief that true empowerment of women and other marginalized human beings begins with the recognition that we all actively participate in the creation of our realities. At present, Carla manages a community counselling program for women who have been abused and their children. She strives to bring heart and spirit to all of her interactions.

INGRID RIVERA, also known as "ING," is a queer, economic and racial justice activist. She was born and raised in Brooklyn, New York, and currently resides there with her ten-year-old daughter and partner. ING has been participating in poetry slams and has been featured at the Nuyorican Poets Café. She has also shared her poetry/spoken word at Bluestockings Woman's Bookstore, Cowpasture Coffee House, DUMBA, and in other venues. She is currently working with the support/funding of Homo-Visiones to develop a Latina-lesbian writers workshop, and she works for the National Gay and Lesbian Task Force-Policy Institute.

ANAKANA GAUGHAN SCHOFIELD came to Canada from Dublin, Ireland, five years ago. She holds a Creative Writing Certificate from Simon Fraser University and was a participant in 2002/3 Banff Wired Writing Studio. She's been published in *Geist* and various anthologies. She recently completed her first novel *The Scuppering of Paudie Mahon* and is raising her four-year-old son Cúán-Isamu.

For the last six years, BELDAN SEZEN spent her days and nights sometimes with writing, performing, teaching, traveling, publishing and (lately) drawing, but most of the times struggling with and enjoying the mysteries of life and love. Turkish, born and raised in Germany, she graduated in political sciences and German linguistics in 1998 and as an animator and story boarder in 2002. She is co-publisher of the anthology *Talking Home – Heimat aus unserer eigenen Feder, women of color in Germany*. Nominated with "ethnic PhD" for the ZAMI-Award 2000 in Amsterdam. Currently she is working as an freelance animator and artist. For further information: *www.homepage.mac.com/beldansezen*

FARAH M. SHROFF, PhD, is an activist, educator, and researcher in the field of public health. She is editor of and contributor to the book *The New Midwifery: Reflections on Renaissance and Regulation* (Women's Press, 1997), as well as other publications in holistic health, women's health HIV/AIDS, social justice, and other areas. She lives in Vancouver with her children and partner.

NEETA SINGH is the recipient of the prestigious Commonwealth Scholarship by the Government of Canada and is currently teaching English literature at Sherubtse College, Bhutan. Her other specific interests are African literature, women's literature, semiotics and Canadian studies. Ms. Singh is also a recipient of the Jawahalal Nehru Memorial Award for her contribution to the field of literature in India, where she obtained her MPhil degree in English literature at the prestigious Jawahalal Nehru University. Ms. Singh has been both a political activist and a freelance journalist in India, which has inspired her to pursue post-colonial studies in Canada. Ms. Singh is interested in studying the effect of marginalization in Canadian society. Neeta has presented widely on women writers like Margaret Atwood, Maria Campbell, and Bessie Head at international conferences and is keen to explore women's literature in cross-cultural terms in Canada. Her comparative approach to literature has proven to be an asset as her work displays a keen understanding of cross-cultural realities and the multicultural experience. Ms. Singh also dabbles in creative writing, theatre, and poetry.

My name is LORRAINE THOMAS. I am thirty-one years old and I am a First Nations Cree. I was born in Prince Albert, Saskatchewan to Amy Thomas (Chamakese) and to George Joseph (Keenamotiayoo). My mother is from the Pelican Lake Reserve and my father is from Big River First Nations Reserve. My adopted uncle dad, through the Aboriginal ways, is Tommy Bear. It is in high esteem that I place my uncle dad Tom Bear alongside my parents. I come from a background of chiefs. I am a descendant of grandfather Good Spirit, on my dad's side. And I am a descendant of Elsie Long Pipe, on my mother's side. I am currently researching my family tree. I am the great-great-granddaughter of Keenamontiayoo of Big River First Nations. I graduated from the University of Saskatchewan in 2003. I graduated with a Bachelor of Education degree from the Indian Teacher Education Program (I.T.E.P.). I am also currently teaching at the Pelican Lake Reserve, SK. My male role model continues to be uncle dad, Lawrence Joseph, who is a vice-chief of the Federation Saskatchewan Indian Nations (F.S.I.N.). I continue to be inspired by my Aboriginal culture. I love and believe in a Creator. I have had several poems published in several anthologies. I currently reside in Leoville, Saskatchewan.

ROXANE TRACEY is a creative writer and visual artist who combines art imagery and poetry in her artwork. The Toronto-based artist seeks to inspire and touch the souls of others with her self-titled Poetic Art. Tracey's artwork has been exhibited in the United States and Canada, and her poetry has been published in various Canadian anthologies.

WENDY VINCENT: I am a thirty-three-year-old Canadian-born single female of proud Jamaican heritage. I've been employed as a Communications Officer at the Canadian Broadcasting Corporation, for the past eight years. I am also a freelance publicist, and my operations specialize in providing publicity for urban musicians and organizations in the black and urban community. My mandate as a publicist is to provide press and buzz for clients who deserve an equal voice in mainstream media. With memberships in the Canadian Association of Black Journalists, the Urban Music Association of Canada, Phem Phat, and the National Association of Black Females in Music and Entertainment, these are busy times! Apart from my invigorated entrepreneurial spirit, I remain vigilant in the care of my reproductive health and am an astute student of black women and fibroids. My myomectomy was a traumatic and defining moment in my life, and I can never revisit those days. I hope my contribution to this anthology will help other black women cope with or avoid what has become a terrible rite of passage for far too many of us. I would like to dedicate this piece to my incredible Vincent and Burton family, my professional family, my support sistahs and brothas and my family to come.

VERA M. WABEGIJIG is Anishnawbe from Ontario. She's a mother. She's a writer. She's creative. She's single. She's short, brown, and loves frybread. Sometimes you can see her opt for natural veggies surrounded by green with frybread on the side. Her mind, her flow, comes with Nish flair but lingering in an urban environment, and sometimes she will forget to make frybread. Her granny taught her to make frybread, and in return she writes in memory of her and all her grannies. Only when she headed west did she find out that there's another word for frybread: bannock. That's east/west flavour.

INGRID WALDRON was born in Montreal, Quebec. She is currently employed as a postdoctoral fellow at the Center for Research in Women's Health at the University of Toronto, where she is conducting research that would allow her to develop an evaluation tool to measure the impact of racism on mental health. She was awarded her PhD degree in 2002 from the Ontario Institute for Studies in Education of the University of Toronto. Her doctoral thesis examines the psychological, emotional, mental, and spiritual impact of oppression on African Canadian women, racism in the history, tradition, and practice of psychiatry, African-centred psychology, and African indigenous knowledge in mental health.

In addition to her academic work, Dr. Waldron has been involved in human rights work locally and internationally for organizations such as COSTI Immigrant Services in Toronto, The Toronto District School Board, and the World Health Organization in Geneva.

PITCHE WASAYANANUNG: I am a First Nations woman on a journey of self-discovery. Through this journey I have learnt much about myself. Counselling is very important along my journey and I now have a support system that I am proud of. I enjoy writing a lot and it opens doorways for me of deeper self-expression. I was taken from my family when I was five years of age. I have spent much of my journey feeling sorry for myself until one day I had enough. I have a nine-year-old daughter who draws her feelings each morning when she gets up. My daughter has PowWow danced since taking her first steps and is very gifted in many ways, I am so proud of my daughter. We live alternatively, growing and eating organic foods; use herbs and homeopathy instead of drugs; do not use chemicals as much as possible yet biodegradable substances; I home school my daughter since she was growing in my body; my daughter was born to midwives with a native ceremony of a hand drum and other gifts from the creator. We both walk the red road as gently and respectfully as possible. I have just taken a Doula training to be a Ceremonial Doula to help the gift of life to start off with ceremonies. I feel ceremonies are deeply missed in our lives today. Our ancestors had a ceremony for everything we did and I feel my journey will help. I encourage everyone to look on the inside if one's life does not feel right. Inner healing is very scary at first yet gets easier as one accepts the process and trusts the creator within us all. Good journey.

CRYSTAL E. WILKINSON is the author of two prize-winning works of fiction. She grew up in rural Kentucky and is a recipient of the Chaffin Award for Appalachian Literature. Her most recent work, Water Street, was a finalist for the Orange Prize and the Zora Neal

Hurston/Richard Wright Legacy Award in Fiction. Her first collection of short stories, *Blackberries, Blackberries* was published by the Toby Press in 2000 to enthusiastic reviews in the regional and national press. She is currently a faculty member of Spalding University's MFA in Writing Program in Louisville, Kentucky.

GITANE WILLIAMS: I am grateful to God for all my blessings and gifts for without Him I am nothing. Growing up in Oakland, California, with the guidance of my mother and the love of all of my family relations, past and present. Today, I am the community activist, the presenter, facilitator, and sometimes wear the hat of the commissioner and the board chair. The prayer counsellor, the sister, the friend of the friendless, all of these I am and can do through Christ who lives in me. Commissioner, Human Welfare and Community Action Commission, City of Berkeley, California, appointed by Council member Kris Worthington, District (7). President, Alameda County Network of Mental Health Clients, Berkeley, Facilitator, Pacific Center for Human Growth, Women's Rap Group, Berkeley. Living my life as a spiritual being in human form, University of Life. PhD (presently here doing it!)

JUDITH K. WITHEROW is a poet, essayist, and storyteller. A mixed blood Native American raised in rural Appalachian poverty, she writes about her life experiences with disability, gender, sexual orientation, race, and class from a perspective influenced by her early heritage. Her work is widely published in scholastic collections, anthologies, and publications directed toward women, lesbians, and native peoples. Her honours include the first annual Audre Lorde Award for non-fiction.

VALERIE WOOD: I am an Ojibway woman who currently resides in Barrie, Ontario, with my partner Mark and our three children, Taylor, Sarah, and Joshua. Writing poetry is not only a creative outlet; it is also cathartic. My family, friends and community are amongst my muses. I have recently discovered the value in the relaxing yet repetitive nature of beading and other craft work. I also find drawing a great way to deal with the daily grind other life struggles. My work with children keeps me young and on my toes and affords me many opportunities to be creative. My family has known the joy of my creativity, as I not only like to cook but experiment in the kitchen as well.